ASHLEY SMITH BIRO

Raising Well-Balanced Kids

A Crunchy Mom's Guide to Natural Health Practices

First edition

This book was professionally typeset on Reedsy.
Find out more at reedsy.com

To my boys, who are my greatest teachers and my endless source of inspiration. Your curiosity, resilience, and boundless love guide me every day.

To my clients, whose trust and journeys have shaped my path and deepened my commitment to holistic health. Your courage and growth remind me why this work matters.

And to the mentors, friends, and kind souls who have shared their wisdom and taught me invaluable lessons along the way—thank you for illuminating my path.

Contents

Foreword

As parents, we all want what's best for our children. We want them to grow up healthy, happy, and equipped with the tools they need to navigate life's challenges with resilience and confidence. But in today's world, it can be overwhelming to know what's truly best. There's so much conflicting information about health, nutrition, wellness, and how to raise well-balanced children. This book is my attempt to share what I've learned on my personal journey as a "crunchy mom" (and in some phases, as even a "scrunchy mom")—embracing a natural, holistic approach to parenting.

I won't lie—sometimes I've picked and chosen what I wanted to believe due to my own limiting belief system. But when I broke down those barriers and opened my mind, I was able to make more informed choices for myself and my children. With all the new information emerging every day, it's nearly impossible to live the perfect, orderly "clean" life. (Actually, I take that back—the Amish do it and do it well. But I am not Amish, nor am I ready to become Amish.) Making the right choices for our families can sometimes be very stressful, but the only way we will make progress as a society is if those of us who identify as "crunchy moms" choose to band together and let our "freak flags" fly.

During my work with Children's Health Defense, I learned a startling statistic: at the rate we're going, there may be no healthy children left in ten years. Luckily, we had already started our crunchy journey, but that statistic scared me. Between the "food" additives (or food-like substances) most of our children are ingesting and the childhood vaccine schedule—which hasn't been properly researched in over 30 years—many children in America are being robbed of their health before they even know what health means.

As the mother of two boys—aged 2 and 13 at the time of this book—I can say my parenting style and choices have evolved dramatically over the past 13 years. When my oldest was born, I trusted the medical system wholeheartedly. We never missed a well- visit. I never questioned my doctor or their recommendations. What they said, went! I was just a mere peasant. What did I know? Phew! Fast-forward 11 years, and I was refusing the pertussis booster during pregnancy, skipping the flu shot, rejecting the COVID vaccine, and even reading my OB the riot act about the blood glucose test during pregnancy. When I finally gave birth to my second son, I opted out of vaccines and wiped the eye ointment off him the moment he was handed to me. (We'll talk more about that in later chapters.) Which child is healthier? 10/10, my youngest. My oldest had a reaction to the MMR vaccine—he ran a high fever, and I'd be willing to say a part of his sweet and bubbly personality disappeared with it. Skyler is still sweet and a very good kid, but he was born with hearing issues, was later diagnosed with sensory processing issues, and spent lots of time with doctors and in therapy. Last August, he was diagnosed as being on the autism spectrum. However, we've decided to raise and treat him like any other child. I absolutely supplemented his diet and cut out pre-packaged foods and dyes many years ago, but originally, my crunchy journey wasn't even for Skyler—it was for me.

In my early twenties, I was diagnosed with lupus after a lifetime of health issues. Although I never tested positive for lupus, doctors routinely suggested that my symptoms presented similarly to it. For years, I followed their advice. I took immunosuppressants and prednisone, but I got worse and worse. I was having intravenous infusions every four weeks, and nothing was working. Eventually, the drug I was on was approved for subcutaneous use! Woohoo! No more spending every fourth Friday in a heated recliner, watching old reruns of *The Young and the Restless* in a room full of elderly arthritis patients. Subcutaneous was a win for me—a true game changer! At the time, I thought I was making healthy choices. I went to the gym daily, chose a healthy Panera sandwich and soup over a cheeseburger, and got enough sleep. It wasn't until the specialty pharmacy sent me the wrong medication that I realized I wasn't okay. I was terrified of what would happen without my meds for four weeks. I fought with the pharmacy, but they weren't going to send the right drug, not for $75,000. I was doomed for an entire month.

Talking with my friend Scott, I learned about Dr. Lauren, a chiropractor and naturopathic doctor in Texas who saw clients virtually. It was expensive, but not $75,000 expensive, so I gave her a shot. I filled out a 26-page intake form—more extensive than anything any doctor had ever asked for—and sent pictures of my tongue, eyes, nails, and more. Dr. Lauren made dietary recommendations, including cutting gluten and sugar, and added a heavy metal detox, fish oil, vitamin D, a high-quality vitamin, and Bach flower remedies. And then I waited. Within four days, all the symptoms I had dealt with for a lifetime—rashes, fevers, and excruciating joint pain—were gone. I was a new woman.

In *Raising Well-Balanced Kids*, I'll share practical tips, natural remedies, and holistic health practices that I've used with my own family. From exploring natural remedies for everyday ailments to finding balance between screen time and outdoor play, this guide is meant to empower you with ideas and strategies that align with a holistic lifestyle. These practices are grounded in my own experiences, my beliefs, and the methods I've found effective for raising children in harmony with nature and health-conscious choices.

That said, this book is not intended to diagnose, treat, or replace professional medical advice. I am not a doctor—I am just a certified holistic health practitioner, a massage and bodywork therapist and a mom with good intentions. The information provided here is purely based on my personal beliefs and experiences as a parent. I encourage you to consult with your healthcare provider before making any significant changes to your child's health regimen, especially if they have underlying medical conditions. Always seek advice from a qualified medical professional when it comes to diagnosing or treating health issues.

The ideas in this book are meant to complement, not replace, the care you may receive from your pediatrician or healthcare provider. I hope you find inspiration and useful tips within these pages, and that you feel empowered to make the best decisions for your family based on your own values and instincts.

Together, let's explore how a natural, holistic approach can support the growth and wellness of the next generation. Welcome to *Raising Well-Balanced Kids*.

1

Embracing the Crunchy Lifestyle

Imagine a world where the pharmacy isn't your first stop when a mild illness hits. Instead of reaching for a bottle of cough syrup or painkillers, you reach for a cup of herbal tea, a tincture, or a natural remedy passed down through generations. For many families, this is not just an ideal—it's the reality they've crafted by choosing to embrace natural health solutions over synthetic alternatives. This chapter is an invitation to discover the "crunchy" lifestyle, a journey toward holistic living that prioritizes wellness, balance, and natural practices for raising well-balanced kids.

The "crunchy mom" approach emphasizes natural health practices as a cornerstone for raising children. It is about aligning with nature, using the body's innate ability to heal, and finding alternatives to conventional medical solutions when appropriate. This chapter introduces the crunchy lifestyle and how it serves as a foundation for raising well-balanced, healthy children in harmony with the natural world.

The Crunchy Mom Mentality

Defining the Lifestyle

The crunchy lifestyle is defined by a commitment to holistic and natural living. It goes beyond simply eating organic foods or using natural products. At its core, it's about honoring the body's ability to heal, prioritizing wellness over convenience, and nurturing a deep connection to the environment. Crunchy moms avoid synthetic chemicals, preservatives, and conventional medications when possible, turning instead to nature's pharmacy. They choose preventive care, like nourishing diets, clean environments, and natural remedies, to support their families' health from the inside out.

The crunchy mentality also encourages education and self-awareness. Crunchy parents tend to ask questions, do research, and trust their instincts when making health decisions for their children. Instead of following the status quo, they often take a proactive approach in learning about alternative health practices, exploring ancient wisdom, and staying open to new approaches that resonate with their values.

Benefits of Steering Away from Conventional Medicine

One of the core principles of the crunchy lifestyle is steering away from conventional medicine as the first resort, especially for minor ailments. Rather than rushing to the pediatrician for every sniffle or scrape, crunchy moms often turn to preventive care and natural remedies to keep their kids healthy. This includes herbal teas, homeopathy, essential oils, and other remedies that support the body's natural healing process.

By choosing this path, parents often find that they rely less on over-the-counter medications and doctor visits for minor issues. Preventive care, such as bolstering the immune system through nutrition, supplements, and healthy habits, becomes a key strategy. Natural remedies for common ailments like colds, fevers, and upset stomachs can be gentler on the body than synthetic medications, which may come with side effects.

While crunchy moms don't entirely reject conventional medicine—there's a time and place for it—they see it as one tool in their health toolbox, rather than the primary solution. They opt for natural solutions first, and when necessary, turn to medical professionals for serious or complex conditions.

Alternative Health Practices for Child Wellness

The crunchy lifestyle embraces a variety of alternative health practices that are often overlooked or misunderstood in conventional medical circles. These approaches, such as iridology, muscle testing, and biofeedback, can offer unique insights into a child's health and wellness, allowing parents to address potential imbalances before they become major issues. In addition to these practices, other holistic methods like herbal medicine, homeopathy, and energy work can further support a child's physical and emotional development.

1. Iridology: Eyes as Windows to Health

Iridology involves examining the patterns, colors, and structures in the iris (the colored part of the eye) to assess overall health and identify areas of the body that may need attention. The idea behind iridology is that the eyes are connected to the body's internal systems, and changes in the iris can reflect underlying health conditions or imbalances.

What Iridology Can Reveal:

- **Digestive Health**: Iridology can help identify potential issues in the digestive tract, such as inflammation or poor nutrient absorption, which are often linked to broader health concerns.

- **Detoxification Needs**: It can also indicate areas where detoxification might be necessary, showing possible liver stress or lymphatic congestion.
- **Inherited Traits**: Iridology can reveal inherited weaknesses or predispositions, allowing parents to take preventative steps to support their child's health.

Iridology: Understanding Health Through the Eyes

Iridology is the study of the iris—the colored part of the eye—to assess a person's health tendencies. Iridologists believe that the iris can reveal information about a person's physical and emotional well-being based on its colors, patterns, and markings. This method does not diagnose diseases but rather provides insights into potential health strengths and weaknesses.

Eye Colors and Their Meanings

1. **Blue or Light-Colored Eyes**:

- Often associated with the lymphatic constitution, which may indicate a tendency toward conditions involving the lymphatic system, respiratory health, or mucous membrane sensitivity.
- Individuals with blue eyes might be more prone to allergies, inflammation, or respiratory issues.

1. **Brown Eyes**:

- Commonly linked to the hematogenic constitution, indicating a potential focus on blood health and digestive functions.

- People with brown eyes may be more likely to experience imbalances related to blood sugar, liver health, and iron levels.

1. **Mixed or Hazel Eyes**:

- Known as the biliary constitution, hazel or mixed-colored eyes can suggest tendencies toward liver and digestive health issues.
- This constitution may show a predisposition to digestive sensitivities, skin issues, and blood sugar fluctuations.

Iris Markings and Their Interpretations

1. **Lacunae (Small Openings or Gaps)**:

- Lacunae are small, leaf-like openings in the iris fibers. They may indicate areas where there could be weaknesses or susceptibilities in specific organs.
- The location of lacunae within different areas of the iris map can suggest which part of the body may need extra support.

1. **Radii Solaris (Radiating Lines)**:

- These are lines that look like rays coming from the pupil outward. They may suggest potential toxicity or digestive sensitivity.
- Radii Solaris can indicate areas in the body that may benefit from detoxification support.

1. **Ring Markings**:

- **Nerve Rings**: Circular rings around the iris may suggest stress and nervous tension. These are often associated with an individual's stress response and may indicate a need for stress management.
- **Scurf Rim**: A dark ring around the edge of the iris, sometimes linked to poor circulation or skin health issues.

1. **Pigment Spots**:

- Pigment spots or dots within the iris can signify metabolic changes or inherited tendencies. The color and location of these pigments may provide additional information about which organs or systems might benefit from support.

Constitution Types in Iridology

Iridology categorizes people into constitutions that highlight genetic strengths and weaknesses. Each constitution gives clues about one's resilience and potential areas of vulnerability, which is determined by how far apart the fibers are in the iris.

Very Resilient Constitution:

- **Characteristics:** Indicates exceptionally strong genetic health and an extremely high level of resilience to stress and illness. The fibers in the iris are very closely packed, showing robust and enduring health. Individuals with this constitution tend to recover rapidly from health challenges and rarely face chronic issues.

Resilient Constitution:

- **Characteristics:** Indicates strong genetic health and overall high resilience to stress and illness. The fibers in the iris are closely packed, showing solid health. Individuals with this constitution often recover quickly from health challenges and have fewer chronic issues.

Mildly Resilient Constitution:

- **Characteristics:** Shows moderate genetic health. The fibers in the iris are moderately spaced, suggesting decent resilience. Individuals may handle stress and illness relatively well but could develop chronic conditions if their lifestyle and environment are not supportive.

Moderately Resilient Constitution:

- **Characteristics:** Indicates an average level of resilience. The iris fibers are more widely spaced compared to resilient constitutions. Individuals may have some inherent weaknesses that require ongoing support and attention to maintain optimal health. They may be more prone to chronic issues if not proactive with their health care.

Using Iridology for Health Insights

Iridology can offer a broad view of your body's unique constitution, highlighting potential areas for strengthening and maintenance. Keep in mind that iridology is not diagnostic but can serve as a complementary tool to gain deeper insights into individual health patterns.

2. Muscle Testing (Applied Kinesiology): Tuning into the Body's Signals

Muscle testing, or applied kinesiology, is a practice that assesses the body's energy and physical responses by evaluating the strength or weakness of specific muscles. It is often used to detect imbalances or sensitivities in the body, guiding parents toward the most appropriate foods, supplements, or remedies for their child's unique needs.

How Muscle Testing Can Be Applied:

- **Nutritional Sensitivities**: Muscle testing can help determine whether a child has sensitivities to certain foods, allowing parents to customize their diet to better support digestion and overall health.
- **Supplementation**: It can also be used to assess which vitamins, minerals, or herbal remedies are most beneficial for a child, ensuring they receive tailored support for their health needs.
- **Emotional and Physical Balance**: Muscle testing is not limited to physical health; it can also provide insights into emotional well-being, helping identify stressors or emotional imbalances that may affect the body.

Step-by-Step Guide to Muscle Reflex Testing for Kids

Before You Begin:

- Find a quiet space with minimal distractions.
- Ensure your child is calm and relaxed.
- Use this method as a tool for general wellness. For serious health concerns, always consult with a healthcare provider.

Step 1: Establish a Baseline Response

1. Position Your Child: Have your child stand up straight, with one arm extended out to the side at shoulder height. Make sure their palm is facing down, and they are standing comfortably with feet flat on the ground.
2. Apply Light Pressure: Stand beside your child and gently place your hand on their extended arm, just above the wrist. Explain to your child that you're going to press down slightly on their arm and that they should resist by trying to keep their arm level.
3. Test the Baseline: Apply light but steady pressure on their arm and ask them to resist as much as they can. This is your baseline for what their arm feels like when their body is strong and in balance.

- Strong Response: The arm stays firm and resists your pressure.
- Weak Response: The arm drops easily under pressure or feels weak.

This step establishes a neutral, balanced state for your child. Now you can use this baseline to test how their body responds to various stimuli.

Step 2: Introduce a Food, Supplement, or Object

1. Hold the Test Item: Place a small amount of food, a supplement, or an object in your child's hand (or hold it against their body, such as near their chest). For example, if you want to test how their body reacts to a certain food, place the food in a small container or in their hand.
2. Repeat the Muscle Test: With the test item in place, ask

your child to extend their arm again. Apply the same amount of pressure as before and ask them to resist your push.

- Positive Response: If the body reacts well to the item, your child's arm should remain strong and resist the pressure, just like in the baseline test.
- Negative Response: If the item is not beneficial for your child, their arm may weaken and drop when you apply pressure.

Example: You can test whether a certain food is causing digestive issues or sensitivity. If their arm weakens when holding the food, it may indicate that their body doesn't respond well to it.

Step 3: Interpret the Results

- Strong Response: A strong, resistant arm indicates that the body is responding positively to the tested item, suggesting it is beneficial or neutral to your child's body.
- Weak Response: A weakened arm or one that drops easily may indicate the tested item is not beneficial for your child, or that their body has an adverse reaction to it.

Repeat the process with other foods, supplements, or environmental factors that you suspect may be affecting your child's health. You can use this method to tailor your child's diet, supplement regimen, or identify sensitivities.

Step 4: Use Muscle Testing for Emotional Well-being

You can also use muscle testing to check for emotional imbalances. Ask your child to think about a situation or feeling that may be causing stress (such as school or friendships). Perform the same muscle test while they focus on the emotion.

- Strong Response: A strong arm indicates they are likely coping well with the emotional situation.
- Weak Response: A weakened arm may suggest that the emotional issue is causing stress or imbalance.

Step 5: Practice Regularly

Muscle reflex testing can be used regularly to check in on your child's health. Whether you're testing foods, supplements, or emotional stressors, it's a useful tool to help ensure your child is in balance. This method is simple, yet it can provide powerful insights into your child's well-being.

Key Points to Remember:

- Be gentle and patient when performing the test.
- Test multiple times to ensure consistent results.
- Muscle testing should be one part of your holistic health toolkit. For more serious or ongoing issues, consult with a healthcare professional.

By following this step-by-step guide, you can empower yourself with a simple, effective tool to support your child's health and wellness. Muscle testing provides real-time feedback from the body, offering insight into how various factors affect their physical and emotional well-being.

3. Biofeedback: Teaching Children to Manage Stress

Biofeedback uses technology to measure physiological responses—such as heart rate, muscle tension, and breathing patterns—and helps individuals learn how to control these processes for better health. This is particularly helpful for children dealing with anxiety, stress, or emotional challenges, as biofeedback teaches them how to self-regulate their body's responses.

Oftentimes biofeedback may be administered by a naturopath, holistic health practitioner or even a chiropractor. Systems to perform biofeedback at home are now readily sold to the public and can be used with a cell phone or home computer.

Benefits of Biofeedback:

- **Stress and Anxiety Reduction**: Biofeedback can be a powerful tool for helping children manage stress and anxiety. By learning to control their physiological responses (like heart rate and breathing), children can develop skills to stay calm in difficult situations.
- **Improved Focus and Attention**: For children with ADHD or attention difficulties, biofeedback can help improve focus and concentration by training the brain to stay more relaxed and alert.
- **Emotional Resilience**: Biofeedback empowers children to understand how their body reacts to emotions, allowing them to manage emotional challenges more effectively.

4. Herbal Medicine: Gentle Support for Growing Bodies

Herbal medicine has been used for centuries to support health and healing in a natural way. For children, herbal remedies can provide gentle, effective support for common issues such as digestive discomfort, colds, and sleep difficulties.

Common Herbal Remedies for Children:

1. Chamomile

- **Uses**: Calming, helps with sleep, soothes digestive issues, and reduces colic.
- **Benefits**: A gentle herb that promotes relaxation and is helpful for easing tummy aches or restlessness in young children. Use as a tea or diluted tincture.

2. Elderberry

- **Uses**: Immune booster, helps with colds and flu.
- **Benefits**: Rich in antioxidants and vitamin C, elderberry syrup is a popular remedy for preventing or reducing the duration of colds and flu.

3. Ginger

- **Uses**: Eases nausea, aids digestion, reduces inflammation.
- **Benefits**: Known for calming upset stomachs, ginger can be used as a tea or diluted syrup, especially effective for motion sickness or digestive discomfort.

4. Echinacea

- **Uses**: Supports immune health, fights off infections.
- **Benefits**: Often used at the onset of cold or flu symptoms, echinacea helps to stimulate the immune system. Best used in short durations.

5. Calendula

- **Uses**: Heals skin irritations, rashes, and minor cuts.
- **Benefits**: Calendula has antibacterial and anti-inflammatory properties, making it ideal for skin issues. Use as a cream or infused oil for cuts, rashes, or diaper rash.

6. Slippery Elm

- **Uses**: Soothes sore throats, coughs, and digestive upset.
- **Benefits**: Its mucilaginous texture coats and soothes irritated mucous membranes. Great for sore throats, coughs, and stomach troubles. Can be used as a powder in teas or lozenges.

7. Fennel

- **Uses**: Eases colic, gas, and digestive discomfort.
- **Benefits**: A mild herb that supports digestion and relieves bloating and gas. Often used in teas for babies and young children with tummy issues.

8. Peppermint

- **Uses**: Calms upset stomachs, eases headaches, and supports respiratory health.
- **Benefits**: Peppermint tea or diluted oil is useful for nausea, colds, and headaches. Its cooling effect helps with fevers and congestion.

9. Lemon Balm

- **Uses**: Calms anxiety, supports sleep, and eases cold sores.
- **Benefits**: Known for its relaxing effects, lemon balm is helpful for reducing anxiety and promoting restful sleep. It can be taken as a tea or diluted tincture.

10. Licorice Root

- **Uses**: Soothes sore throats, reduces coughing, and aids digestion.
- **Benefits**: With soothing and anti-inflammatory properties, licorice root is great for respiratory issues and digestive discomfort. Use as a tea or syrup for older children.

Usage Tips

- **Forms**: These herbs are typically used as teas, syrups, or diluted tinctures.
- **Dosage**: Follow age-appropriate guidelines or consult a healthcare provider, as children's dosages differ from adults.

These herbal remedies provide gentle, effective support for common childhood issues like colds, upset stomachs, and skin irritations, making them ideal for any holistic family toolkit.

5. Homeopathy: Tailored Remedies for Individual Needs

Homeopathy is a gentle, natural system of medicine that uses highly diluted substances to stimulate the body's healing response. It can be particularly effective for children, as it addresses the body's imbalances without the side effects that can come with conventional medicine.

Common Homeopathic Remedies for Children:

1. Chamomilla

- **Uses**: Teething pain, irritability, restlessness, and colic.
- **Description**: Ideal for children who become very irritable, especially during teething, and may seem inconsolable.

2. Arnica Montana

- **Uses**: Bruises, muscle soreness, bumps, and falls.
- **Description**: Known for its ability to reduce pain and swelling; great for treating bumps and bruises from minor accidents.

3. Pulsatilla

- **Uses**: Colds, clinginess, earaches, and emotional sensitivity.
- **Description**: Especially useful for children who seek comfort when unwell and are prone to weepy or clingy behavior.

4. Belladonna

- **Uses**: High fever, sore throat, earaches, and headaches.
- **Description**: Suitable for children with sudden-onset symptoms, particularly fevers that come with a flushed face.

5. Aconitum Napellus (Aconite)

- **Uses**: Sudden fever, colds, shock, and anxiety after a scare.
- **Description**: Helpful in the early stages of illness, especially after exposure to cold wind or a sudden fright.

6. Nux Vomica

- **Uses**: Digestive issues, stomach pain, constipation, and irritability.
- **Description**: For children with stomach troubles, especially after overeating or eating foods that are difficult to digest.

7. Ferrum Phosphoricum

- **Uses**: Early stages of fever, mild infections, colds, and flu symptoms.
- **Description**: Great for early-onset illnesses, especially when there's low-grade fever and general fatigue.

8. Calcarea Phosphorica

- **Uses**: Growing pains, bone development, teething issues.
- **Description**: A supportive remedy for children experiencing rapid growth or discomfort related to bone and teeth development.

9. Silicea

- **Uses**: Abscesses, skin conditions, and boosting immunity.
- **Description**: Helpful for children prone to skin eruptions, weak immunity, or those with trouble healing from minor wounds.

10. Bryonia

- **Uses**: Coughs, colds, body aches, and flu-like symptoms.

- **Description**: For dry, painful coughs or colds with body aches, especially when movement makes symptoms worse.

Usage Notes

- **Dilution**: Homeopathic remedies are often given in 6C or 30C potency for children.
- **Dosage**: Generally, 2-3 pellets dissolved under the tongue or in a small amount of water. Follow dosage instructions on the remedy or as advised by a healthcare professional.

These remedies provide gentle, supportive care for common childhood ailments and can be a valuable addition to your holistic toolkit.

6. Energy Medicine: Balancing Body and Mind

Energy medicine, including practices like Reiki and healing touch, focuses on balancing the body's energy systems to promote healing and wellness. For children, these gentle, non-invasive therapies can be particularly effective in calming the nervous system and supporting emotional well-being.

Benefits of Energy Medicine for Children:

- **Calming and Grounding**: Energy medicine practices can help highly sensitive or anxious children feel more grounded and calm, promoting emotional stability.
- **Support During Illness**: These therapies can also support the body's natural healing processes during illness, helping children recover more quickly from common ailments.
- **Emotional Healing**: Energy healing can address emotional blockages that may manifest as physical symptoms, provid-

ing holistic support for both body and mind.

10-Step At-Home Energy Work Guide for Parents and Kids

Step 1: Prepare the Space

- **How**: Create a calming environment by dimming the lights, playing soft music, or lighting a candle.
- **Purpose**: Establishes a relaxing space that encourages a sense of safety and comfort.

Step 2: Set an Intention

- **How**: Begin by setting a gentle intention for the session, such as "calm and balance" or "peace and relaxation."
- **Purpose**: Helps focus your energy and aligns your intention with a positive outcome for your child.

Step 3: Center Yourself

- **How**: Take a few deep breaths to ground and center yourself. Visualize any tension releasing as you exhale.
- **Purpose**: Prepares you to be fully present, calm, and focused during the session.

Step 4: Place Hands on Crown

- **How**: Lightly place your hands on the top of your child's head, allowing energy to flow to the crown.
- **Purpose**: Balances the crown chakra and helps your child feel safe and connected.

Step 5: Move to Forehead and Brow (Third Eye)

- **How**: Gently place your hands over your child's forehead, above the eyes.
- **Purpose**: Soothes the mind, supports relaxation, and may enhance focus and clarity.

Step 6: Place Hands on Shoulders

- **How**: Lightly rest your hands on each shoulder.
- **Purpose**: Provides a calming sense of grounding and stability, relieving any emotional burdens.

Step 7: Heart Center

- **How**: Place your hands on your child's chest, over the heart area.
- **Purpose**: Supports emotional well-being, encourages love and security, and promotes emotional balance.

Step 8: Solar Plexus (Upper Abdomen)

- **How**: Move your hands to the upper abdomen, just below the rib cage.
- **Purpose**: Calms the "butterflies" or stress in the stomach area, supporting confidence and personal strength.

Step 9: Hands on Knees or Lower Abdomen

- **How**: Place hands gently on your child's knees or lower abdomen.

- **Purpose**: Grounds the body, promoting a sense of physical stability and security.

Step 10: Finish with Feet

- **How**: Place your hands lightly on each foot, allowing any remaining tension or energy to flow out.
- **Purpose**: Releases remaining energy blockages, grounding the body and providing closure to the session.

Closing and Gratitude

End the session by gently lifting your hands away. Thank your child and the energy for their openness, encouraging them to take a few deep breaths.

A Holistic Approach to Child Wellness

These alternative health practices offer a comprehensive, holistic approach to understanding and supporting your child's wellness. From iridology and muscle testing to biofeedback and herbal medicine, these tools help parents get to the root of health issues and create personalized wellness plans that cater to each child's unique needs. By embracing these practices, you can foster a deeper connection to your child's health and provide them with the resources they need to thrive naturally.

A Personal Journey: Transitioning from Pharmaceuticals to Holistic Practices

For many crunchy moms, the journey toward holistic health starts with frustration—frustration with conventional medicine's "one-size-fits-all" approach, or with the side effects their children experience from pharmaceuticals. Part of our journey began when my child had recurring ear infections. Even after multiple sets of tubes which caused scarring in the ear canal and even permanent t-tubes, we struggled. Each time, we were prescribed antibiotics, but the infections kept returning. That's when I started researching natural alternatives. I learned about garlic oil ear drops, dietary changes, and chiropractic adjustments that could prevent ear infections in the first place. Slowly, we started relying less on prescriptions and more on nature. It wasn't an overnight transformation, but with every step, I saw improvements in my child's health and well-being. This experience opened the door to a whole new world of natural health practices that I've embraced ever since.

Real-Life Examples of Crunchy Moms

There are countless stories of mothers who have embraced the crunchy lifestyle and seen measurable improvements in their children's health. Take Sarah, for instance, a mom of two who dealt with chronic eczema in her youngest child. After months of using steroid creams prescribed by her pediatrician with little improvement, Sarah decided to seek out alternative solutions. She saw me for a holistic health consultation. We were able to triangulate foods that might be affecting her child's skin through muscle testing, biofeedback and looking at a food journal and comparing self reported symptoms. She switched to a clean, natural diet, eliminating processed foods and allergens, and introduced herbal remedies to support her child's skin health. Over time, the eczema cleared up completely, and Sarah realized the power of nutrition and natural care in promoting lasting wellness.

Then there's Maria, a mom who incorporated muscle testing

into her routine for identifying food sensitivities in her children. By understanding which foods triggered behavioral issues and digestive discomfort, she was able to make informed dietary changes that drastically improved her kids' well-being. These stories reflect the flexibility, curiosity, and dedication that define the crunchy lifestyle.

A crunchy lifestyle is about making conscious choices for your family's health. It's about choosing natural remedies, alternative health practices, and preventive care that promote balance and wellness in your children. By embracing this lifestyle, you're not just treating symptoms—you're supporting your child's overall well-being from the inside out.

Crunchy Pregnancy Choices: Embracing Natural Birth Practices

Pregnancy is a time when many parents start to explore more natural, holistic approaches to health. Making informed decisions during pregnancy can set the foundation for a natural lifestyle that carries into parenthood. In this section, we'll explore common pregnancy interventions, such as the blood glucose test, pertussis booster, and routine newborn procedures, and discuss crunchy alternatives that empower parents to choose what's best for their families.

1. The Blood Glucose Test: An Alternative Approach

The glucose tolerance test, commonly administered between 24-28 weeks of pregnancy, screens for gestational diabetes. However, some mothers prefer to avoid the high-sugar drink used during this test, which can feel overwhelming, especially for those committed to natural living.

Crunchy Alternative: Self-Monitoring Blood Glucose

Instead of the glucose drink, you can ask your healthcare provider for the option to monitor your blood sugar levels at home for one to two weeks. This involves checking your blood sugar at different times throughout the day using a glucometer, particularly after meals. This method provides a more accurate reflection of how your body processes real foods, rather than a large dose of glucose in one sitting.

Why it's a good option:

- Avoids unnecessary sugar intake.
- Provides a more realistic picture of how your body manages blood sugar levels on a daily basis.

2. Declining the Pertussis Booster and Other Vaccinations During Pregnancy

The Tdap vaccine (tetanus, diphtheria, and pertussis) is often recommended during pregnancy to protect newborns from whooping cough. However, some parents choose to decline the pertussis booster due to concerns about vaccine safety or prefer to build their baby's immunity naturally through breastfeeding and delayed exposure.

Why some crunchy moms refuse the booster:

- **Natural Immunity**: Many mothers believe that breastfeeding offers a natural way to transfer immunity to the baby. The colostrum (first milk) is particularly rich in antibodies, helping to protect the newborn's immune system.
- **Minimal Exposure**: By practicing safe exposure methods and limiting contact with potentially sick individuals in the early weeks, you can reduce the risk of pertussis naturally.
- **Risk Factor**: The CDC ordered that pregnant women begin

to get the Pertussis booster while pregnant during 2011. The practice of administering the flu vaccine during any trimester began in 2004. The FDA is responsible for vaccine safety and licensing, but in multiple court documents, admits that it has no safety data to back up the CDC's "off-license" pregnancy recommendations. FDA's website states that it has never formally approved any vaccines "specifically for use during pregnancy to protect the infant." CDC data show that women who received certain flu shots from 2010 to 2012 had a 7.7 times greater risk of miscarriage than women who did not receive those vaccines. (Source: Bono, Lauren. 11 February 2019. FDA Admits That Government Is Recommending Untested, Unlicensed Vaccines for Pregnant Women. Found online at https://childrenshealthdefense.org/news/fda-admits-that-government-is-recommending-untested-unlicensed-vaccines-for-pregnant-women/.)

3. Refusing the Vitamin K Shot at Time of Birth

Vitamin K is typically administered via an injection at birth to help blood clot properly and prevent hemorrhagic disease in newborns. However, some crunchy parents decline this shot and instead opt for natural methods of boosting their baby's vitamin K levels. Most hospitals do require the Vitamin K shot at time of birth in the event that you plan to circumcise your child.

Crunchy Alternative: Oral Vitamin K or Dietary Supplementation

For parents who are concerned about the synthetic ingredients in the injection, oral vitamin K drops are an alternative that can be given to the baby over the first few weeks of life. Another option is ensuring the mother consumes vitamin K-rich foods during pregnancy, such as leafy greens, to naturally support the baby's levels after birth.

Reasons some moms refuse the shot:

- **Dietary Support**: If the mother's diet is rich in vitamin K, the baby may naturally receive sufficient levels through breastfeeding.
- **Preference for Oral Administration**: Some parents prefer a slower, more natural approach using oral vitamin K drops instead of a one-time injection.

4. Refusing Eye Ointment for Newborns

Erythromycin eye ointment is commonly applied to newborns to prevent eye infections caused by bacteria present during birth. However, many crunchy parents opt out of this intervention, especially if they've had a low-risk pregnancy with no signs of infection.

Why it's often not necessary:

- **Low Risk of Infection**: For parents who have tested negative for sexually transmitted infections, the risk of the baby contracting an eye infection is minimal, making the ointment unnecessary.
- **Natural Bonding**: Refusing the ointment allows for uninterrupted eye contact between mother and baby immediately after birth, which supports bonding and attachment.
- **Reducing Unnecessary Antibiotic Exposure:** May contribute to the growing issue of antibiotic resistance and interruptions to the normal flora in the body—a journey best avoided from day one.

5. Refusing Other Routine Shots at Birth

In many hospitals, vaccines such as hepatitis B are offered within the first 24 hours of a baby's life.This is unnecessary since most mothers are not iv drug or needle users, reside in homes with iv needle users and the infant in question does not use drugs or needles. Some crunchy parents prefer to delay or refuse these vaccinations, feeling that newborns should not be exposed to vaccines so early without a clear medical necessity.

Why some parents choose to wait:

- **Delay for Immune Maturity**: Some believe that delaying vaccines until the child's immune system is more developed allows for a stronger, more natural immune response.
- **Breastfeeding Support**: By breastfeeding, mothers can pass on immunity to their babies, reducing the need for immediate vaccines at birth.
- **Acute Infection:** Hepatitis B is treated in most cases as an acute infection and walk away with immunity.
- **Toxicity**: The vaccine uses aluminum as the CDC definition of an "antigen" to create an immune response and contains another neurotoxin, Mercury.
- **Unethical Creation of the Vaccine:** Just look up the Willowbrook State School in New York and Hepatitis B. Enough said.

The Debate on Circumcision: Weighing the Choices

Circumcision is a practice that has been debated for decades, with strong opinions on both sides. For parents making this decision, understanding the arguments for and against circumcision is essential for making an informed choice that aligns with their beliefs and their child's well-being.

Arguments for Circumcision

- **Hygiene and Health Benefits**: Proponents argue that circumcision can make hygiene easier, potentially reducing the risk of infections and conditions like balanitis (inflammation of the foreskin).
- **Medical Prevention**: Some studies suggest circumcision may lower the risk of certain sexually transmitted infections (STIs) and urinary tract infections (UTIs) during infancy.
- **Cultural and Religious Traditions**: In many cultures and religions, circumcision is a significant rite of passage that holds deep meaning.

Arguments Against Circumcision

- **Ethical Considerations**: Critics point to the ethical question of performing an irreversible procedure on a child who cannot consent, emphasizing the right to bodily autonomy.
- **Medical Risks**: Although the risks are relatively low, circumcision can result in complications such as infection, excessive bleeding, and, in rare cases, more serious outcomes.
- **Potential Loss of Sensitivity**: Some argue that circumcision can lead to reduced sensitivity in adulthood, though this point is still debated among medical professionals.

Holistic Considerations

For families following a holistic path, the decision often comes down to weighing the medical, ethical, and cultural aspects. Parents may consider non-surgical options for hygiene and infection prevention or delay the decision until their child is old enough to provide input.

Trusting Your Instincts During Pregnancy

Choosing natural, holistic approaches to pregnancy and birth can empower parents to feel more in control of their family's health decisions. By opting for alternatives like monitoring blood sugar levels instead of the glucose test, or declining interventions such as the pertussis booster, vitamin K shot, and eye ointment, you can align your pregnancy and birth choices with your commitment to a crunchy, natural lifestyle.

How Crunchy Are You?

Take this quiz to see how deep into the "crunchy" lifestyle you are! For each question, choose the answer that best reflects your current habits. Add up your points at the end to find out your score.

1. When it comes to food, your family mostly eats...

A) Whatever is convenient (takeout, processed snacks) – 1 point
B) A mix of whole foods and processed foods – 2 points
C) Mostly whole, organic, and homemade meals – 3 points

2. When your child has a mild cold or fever, you...

A) Reach for over-the-counter medicine – 1 point
B) Use a mix of natural remedies and conventional medicine – 2 points
C) Opt for herbal teas, essential oils, and rest – 3 points

3. How do you clean your home?

A) With conventional, store-bought cleaners – 1 point

B) A mix of natural and conventional products – 2 points

C) DIY natural cleaners like vinegar, baking soda, and essential oils – 3 points

4. Your views on vaccinations are...

A) I follow the standard schedule without question – 1 point

B) I've done some research and selectively vaccinate – 2 points

C) I've thoroughly researched alternatives and take a natural approach – 3 points

5. When it comes to skincare for your family, you use...

A) Whatever is on sale or recommended by ads – 1 point

B) Some natural products, but also drugstore brands – 2 points

C) Organic or DIY skincare with simple, natural ingredients – 3 points

6. How do you approach dental care?

A) Conventional toothpaste and dental products – 1 point

B) A mix of conventional and natural products – 2 points

C) Natural toothpaste (DIY or fluoride-free) and oil pulling – 3 points

7. What's your stance on household products?

A) I don't really think about it – 1 point

B) I'm switching to some non-toxic options – 2 points

C) I've replaced almost all household items with non-toxic, Eco-friendly products – 3 points

8. When it comes to baby care products, you...

A) Use what's most popular or recommended – 1 point

B) Look for gentle options but don't stress over every ingredient – 2 points

C) Use only organic, chemical-free baby products – 3 points

9. How do you view conventional medicine?

A) I trust doctors and follow their advice without question – 1 point

B) I prefer to blend conventional medicine with natural remedies – 2 points

C) I rely mostly on alternative health practices like herbs, homeopathy, and holistic therapies – 3 points

10. What's your approach to clothing?

A) Whatever is stylish and affordable – 1 point

B) I try to avoid fast fashion but still buy conventional brands – 2 points

C) I choose organic, Eco-friendly fabrics or secondhand clothes – 3 points

What's Your Crunch Factor?

10-15 Points: Just Starting the Crunchy Journey

You're curious about natural health but still lean on conventional practices. That's okay! There's always room to grow, and embracing a crunchy lifestyle is a gradual process.

16-23 Points: On the Way to Crunchy

You've already embraced several holistic health principles but still mix in some conventional habits. Keep exploring natural health practices—you're well on your way!

24-30 Points: Super Crunchy

You're living the full crunchy lifestyle! From natural remedies to Eco-friendly products, you prioritize holistic, natural solutions for nearly every aspect of life.

Guide to Finding a Healthcare Provider That Complements Your Health Choices

Choosing a healthcare provider who respects and supports your natural, holistic approach is essential to maintaining consistency in your family's health journey. Whether you're looking for a pediatrician, naturopath, or holistic practitioner, it's important to find someone who aligns with your values and complements your health choices.

Here's how to find a provider that works with you, not against you:

Step 1: Define What You're Looking For

Before starting your search, clearly define the type of healthcare you want for your family. Ask yourself these questions:

- Do I want a provider who is open to alternative therapies like homeopathy, herbal medicine, or acupuncture?
- How important is it that my provider respects my stance on vaccines, medications, or supplements?
- Do I need someone who offers a blend of conventional and holistic approaches (integrative medicine), or do I prefer someone fully focused on natural health?
- Am I seeking specialized care for specific conditions, such as a naturopath for chronic issues or a chiropractor for physical health?

Being clear on your expectations will help guide your search and set the tone for conversations with potential providers.

Step 2: Use Holistic Health Networks and Directories

There are various resources available for finding healthcare providers who practice holistic, integrative, or natural medicine. Some trusted sources include:

- **Holistic Health Directories**: Websites like the **Institute for Functional Medicine**, **American Association of Naturopathic Physicians**, and **National Certification Commission for Acupuncture and Oriental Medicine** provide directories of certified practitioners who offer holistic care.
- **Word of Mouth and Online Communities**: Crunchy parenting groups on social media or holistic health forums are great places to ask for recommendations. Parents often share their experiences with providers who support alternative health choices.
- **Health Food Stores and Wellness Centers**: Many natural health stores and wellness centers have referral lists or in-house practitioners who specialize in holistic care. This can be a great starting point.

Step 3: Conduct a Pre-Screening

Once you have a list of potential providers, it's important to do some initial research. You can usually find out about a provider's philosophy by checking their website, reading reviews, or calling the office to ask a few basic questions. Some questions to consider:

- **Do they have experience with alternative therapies?**
- **Do they respect parental choice when it comes to vaccines,**

medications, or supplements?

- **What's their approach to preventive care?** (Do they emphasize lifestyle, nutrition, and natural remedies?)
- **How open are they to working with other holistic practitioners?**

Step 4: Schedule a Meet-and-Greet or Appointment to Establish Care

Before committing to a provider, it's important to meet them in person. Many healthcare providers offer free consultations or short appointments to get to know you and answer your questions. This is an excellent opportunity to assess their attitude, openness, and communication style. Some may require you to establish care with a physical.

Questions to Ask During the Visit:

- **What is your approach to preventive care?** You want to hear an emphasis on lifestyle factors like nutrition, sleep, and natural therapies.
- **Are you comfortable with parents who choose not to follow the standard vaccination schedule or who prefer alternative treatments?** A supportive provider will respect your choices, even if they don't necessarily agree with them.
- **How do you feel about integrating holistic or complementary therapies, like herbal medicine, homeopathy, or acupuncture, into your treatment plans?** This question helps assess their openness to working with a holistic framework.
- **Do you offer (or refer out for) services like acupuncture, biofeedback, chiropractic care, or nutritional counseling?**

Providers with a network of holistic resources are often more supportive of natural approaches.

Step 5: Evaluate Communication and Respect

After meeting the provider, evaluate how you felt about the interaction:

- **Did they listen to your concerns without judgment?**
- **Did they take the time to understand your perspective and answer your questions thoroughly?**
- **Did they seem open to working with you to create a plan that reflects your family's health values?**

A provider who listens carefully and respects your choices is key to a successful partnership. If you feel pressured, judged, or dismissed, it may be a sign to keep looking.

Step 6: Trust Your Gut

Ultimately, the right provider should make you feel comfortable, respected, and empowered. If you feel confident that the provider will work with you rather than against you, trust your gut instinct and move forward. If something feels off, it's okay to continue your search until you find a better fit.

Where to Look for Holistic Providers

Here are a few types of healthcare providers that may align with natural health choices:

- **Naturopathic Doctors (NDs)**: NDs focus on using natural remedies and therapies to treat health issues. They emphasize prevention, nutrition, and lifestyle changes.

- **Integrative or Functional Medicine Practitioners**: These providers combine conventional and alternative approaches to create personalized treatment plans that focus on the root cause of illness.
- **Chiropractors**: Chiropractors emphasize spinal health and holistic healing, often offering natural therapies like nutrition counseling and supplements.
- **Holistic Pediatricians**: Pediatricians who are open to integrative or alternative treatments and respect parental choice when it comes to vaccines or medication.

Finding the Right Provider for Your Family

Finding a healthcare provider who aligns with your holistic health choices requires patience and research, but it's worth the effort to build a trusted partnership. By clearly defining your health priorities, asking the right questions, and trusting your instincts, you can find a provider who complements your approach to raising well-balanced, naturally healthy kids.

This chapter has introduced the crunchy lifestyle and how it offers parents alternative options for health care, encouraging a shift toward natural, conscious parenting. By trusting in nature's ability to heal and taking proactive steps to support your child's health, you can raise well-balanced, healthy kids who thrive in harmony with the world around them.

Next, we'll dive deeper into one of the foundational aspects of natural health: understanding food as medicine. In the next chapter, we'll explore how nutrition plays a vital role in raising well-balanced children and how food choices can serve as powerful tools for wellness.

2

Food as Medicine

In the 1940s, during the turmoil of wartime, food shortages made clear how crucial food is not only for survival but also for sustaining health. Families were forced to rethink their diets, making do with what was available. This period revealed a profound truth: food is more than just fuel—it's medicine. It has the power to heal, nourish, and sustain life in ways that go far beyond filling empty stomachs. This chapter will explore how food, when chosen wisely and with intention, can be a powerful tool for raising well-balanced, healthy children.

Nutrition is the foundation of health, and understanding food as medicine is a key principle in the crunchy lifestyle. By nourishing children with nutrient-dense, whole foods, we can support not just their physical growth but also their cognitive, emotional, and behavioral development. This chapter will dive into the role of nutrition in promoting overall wellness, illustrating how food choices serve as preventive medicine in the holistic approach to parenting.

The Benefits of Breastfeeding

Breastfeeding offers unparalleled nutritional benefits and provides the foundation for optimal growth and development during infancy. Not only is breast milk the most natural and complete food source for a baby, but it also delivers vital nutrients in a form that is easily digestible. Additionally, breastfeeding supports both the physical and emotional bond between mother and child, fostering lifelong health benefits for both.

Nutritional Benefits of Breastfeeding

- **Complete Nutrition**: Breast milk contains the perfect balance of proteins, fats, vitamins, and carbohydrates needed for a baby's growth. It naturally adapts to meet the changing needs of the growing infant, from colostrum in the early days (rich in antibodies and protein) to mature milk full of essential fats and calories.
- **Immunity Boost**: Breast milk is packed with antibodies that protect babies from infections and illnesses. These antibodies are crucial in the first months of life when a baby's immune system is still developing. Breastfed babies tend to have a lower risk of respiratory infections, gastrointestinal issues, and ear infections.
- **Healthy Gut Development**: Breast milk promotes the growth of healthy gut bacteria, supporting digestion and reducing the risk of gastrointestinal issues. It also helps protect against conditions like colic and constipation.

Long-Term Health Benefits

- **Reduced Risk of Chronic Diseases**: Studies show that breastfeeding reduces the risk of chronic conditions later in life, including obesity, type 2 diabetes, and heart disease. The balanced nutrition in breast milk helps regulate growth and metabolism in infancy, which carries long-term benefits.
- **Cognitive Development**: Breastfeeding has been linked to enhanced brain development and higher cognitive function. The fatty acids in breast milk, particularly DHA, play a key role in the development of the brain and nervous system.
- **Bonding and Emotional Benefits**: Beyond the nutritional value, breastfeeding fosters a strong emotional bond be-

tween mother and child. The close contact, skin-to-skin connection, and hormonal release during breastfeeding support the emotional well being of both mother and baby. This connection can reduce stress and promote healthy emotional development in infants.

Benefits for Mothers

- **Postpartum Recovery**: Breastfeeding helps the mother's body recover more quickly from childbirth by stimulating uterine contractions, which reduces postpartum bleeding. It also promotes the release of oxytocin, which aids in emotional bonding and reduces the risk of postpartum depression.
- **Lowered Risk of Disease**: Breastfeeding has been shown to reduce the mother's risk of breast and ovarian cancers, as well as type 2 diabetes. The extended benefits of breastfeeding protect both mother and child well beyond infancy.

Principles of Whole Food Nutrition

In today's fast-paced world, convenience often takes precedence over nutrition. But when we return to the basics—whole, unprocessed foods—we reconnect with the simple truth that what we feed our children shapes their health, behavior, and overall development. The goal of whole food nutrition is to provide the body with essential nutrients that support growth and balance, while avoiding the synthetic additives, preservatives, and processed ingredients that can harm long-term health.

Nutrient-Dense Foods for Growth

The concept of nutrient density is simple: some foods provide a higher concentration of vitamins, minerals, and beneficial compounds than others. These foods, often whole and unprocessed, are packed with the nutrients children need for optimal growth and development. Foods like leafy greens, fruits, whole grains, legumes, and high-quality proteins form the foundation of a healthy, balanced diet.

Incorporating nutrient-dense foods into a child's diet doesn't need to be complicated. Here are some key elements:

Leafy Greens (Spinach, Kale): Loaded with vitamins A, C, K, iron, and calcium, greens are essential for bone and immune health.

- **How to Disguise**: Blend spinach or kale into smoothies with berries and bananas to mask the taste, or add finely chopped greens to sauces, soups, or scrambled eggs.

Berries (Blueberries, Strawberries, Raspberries): High in antioxidants and vitamin C, these fruits help boost immunity and support brain health.

- **How to Disguise**: Add berries to yogurt parfaits, mix them into muffins or pancakes, or freeze them for a sweet, ice-cream-like treat.

Whole Grains (Quinoa, Brown Rice, Oats): Rich in fiber and B vitamins, whole grains provide energy and enhance cognitive function.

- **How to Disguise**: Make kid-friendly quinoa "fried rice" with veggies, add oats to smoothies for a creamy texture, or turn brown rice into a tasty stir-fry with their favorite proteins.

Healthy Fats (Avocados, Almonds, Chia Seeds): Essential for brain development and hormone balance.

- **How to Disguise**: Blend avocado into smoothies for a creamy texture, make chocolate avocado pudding, or sprinkle chia seeds into yogurt or muffins for an extra boost.

Lean Proteins (Beans, Salmon, Organic Chicken): Providing amino acids necessary for muscle growth and repair.

- **How to Disguise**: Try adding beans to taco fillings, make salmon or chicken patties with fun dipping sauces, or sneak finely chopped chicken or beans into quesadillas and wraps.

By incorporating these foods regularly into meals, you can ensure that your child's diet is filled with the nutrients they need to thrive. Avoiding highly processed foods, refined sugars, and artificial additives can make a significant difference in their overall health and behavior.

10 Kid Friendly Recipes

1. Berry Spinach Smoothie Bowl

- **Ingredients**: 1 cup mixed berries, 1 handful spinach, 1 banana, 1/2 cup Greek yogurt, 1/2 cup almond milk, 1 tbsp chia seeds.
- **Directions**: Blend berries, spinach, banana, yogurt, and almond milk until smooth. Pour into a bowl and top with sliced bananas, more berries, and a sprinkle of chia seeds.

2. Quinoa Veggie "Fried Rice"

- **Ingredients**: 1 cup cooked quinoa, 1/2 cup peas and carrots, 1 scrambled egg, 1 tbsp soy sauce, 1 tbsp olive oil, 1/4 cup finely chopped spinach or kale.
- **Directions**: Saute peas, carrots, and spinach in olive oil. Add quinoa and soy sauce, stirring in the scrambled egg last. Serve as a flavorful, nutrient-packed side or main dish.

3. Mini Avocado & Berry Toasts

- **Ingredients**: 1 ripe avocado, 1 cup mixed berries, 4 slices whole-grain bread, a drizzle of honey.
- **Directions**: Toast the bread, mash avocado, and spread it over the toast. Top with berries and drizzle with a bit of honey. Kids will love the bright colors and mix of textures!

4. Chicken & Spinach Quesadilla

- **Ingredients**: 1 cup shredded cooked chicken, 1/2 cup shredded cheese, 1/4 cup finely chopped spinach, 2 whole-grain tortillas.
- **Directions**: Layer chicken, cheese, and spinach between the tortillas. Cook in a skillet until golden brown, then cut into triangles for an easy-to-eat snack.

5. Hidden Veggie Mac & Cheese

- **Ingredients**: 1 cup whole-grain pasta, 1/2 cup shredded cheddar cheese, 1/4 cup steamed cauliflower, 1/4 cup chopped spinach, 1/4 cup milk.

- **Directions**: Blend cauliflower, spinach, and milk until smooth. Pour over cooked pasta, add cheese, and stir until melted. This cheesy pasta hides nutritious greens and cauliflower for extra veggies.

6. *Banana Berry Oatmeal Muffins*

- **Ingredients**: 1 cup rolled oats, 1/2 cup whole-wheat flour, 1/2 cup mashed banana, 1/2 cup berries, 1/4 cup honey, 1 egg, 1 tsp baking powder.
- **Directions**: Mix all ingredients, fold in berries, and pour batter into a muffin tin. Bake at 350°F for 20 minutes. Great for breakfast or an on-the-go snack.

7. *Salmon & Sweet Potato Patties*

- **Ingredients**: 1 can salmon, 1/2 cup mashed sweet potato, 1 egg, 1/4 cup finely chopped spinach, 1/4 cup breadcrumbs.
- **Directions**: Mix ingredients, form into small patties, and cook in a lightly oiled skillet. Serve with a side of yogurt dipping sauce for extra fun.

8. *Veggie & Chicken Stir-Fry with Brown Rice*

- **Ingredients**: 1 cup cooked brown rice, 1/2 cup chopped chicken, 1/2 cup mixed veggies (carrots, bell peppers, broccoli), 1 tbsp soy sauce, 1 tsp sesame oil.
- **Directions**: Saute veggies and chicken until cooked, add soy sauce, then stir in the brown rice. A colorful, balanced meal packed with protein and fiber.

9. Chia Seed Yogurt Parfait

- **Ingredients**: 1 cup Greek yogurt, 1 tbsp chia seeds, 1/2 cup mixed berries, 1 tbsp honey, granola (optional).
- **Directions**: Layer yogurt with chia seeds, berries, and honey. Top with granola if desired. Kids can help layer their own parfait, making it a fun and nutritious breakfast or snack.

10. Spinach & Cheese Stuffed Turkey Meatballs

- **Ingredients**: 1/2 lb ground turkey, 1/4 cup finely chopped spinach, 1/4 cup shredded cheese, 1/4 cup breadcrumbs, 1 egg.
- **Directions**: Mix turkey, spinach, cheese, breadcrumbs, and egg. Form into small meatballs and bake at 375°F for 20 minutes. Serve with a side of marinara sauce for dipping.

Suggested Caloric Intakes for Children

Understanding caloric needs can help ensure children receive the energy and nutrients required for healthy growth. The following ranges are based on guidelines from the USDA and the American Academy of Pediatrics, providing general targets to support balanced development. Individual needs may vary depending on activity level, growth rate, and unique health factors.

- **Toddlers (1-3 years)**: 1,000–1,400 calories/day
- **Young Children (4-8 years)**: 1,200–1,800 calories/day
- **Preteens (9-13 years)**: 1,600–2,200 calories/day for girls, 1,800–2,600 calories/day for boys

- **Teenagers (14-18 years)**: 1,800–2,400 calories/day for girls, 2,200–3,200 calories/day for boys

These caloric ranges reflect averages across age groups and activity levels, offering a framework to help parents plan balanced, whole-food-based diets. A diet rich in fruits, vegetables, whole grains, lean proteins, and healthy fats is recommended to support these needs effectively.

Diet's Effect on Behavior and Learning

It's easy to overlook the profound connection between diet and a child's behavior or learning capacity. However, the foods we give our children have a direct impact on how they feel, think, and behave. For instance, blood sugar regulation plays a huge role in maintaining a child's mood and focus. Sugary snacks, processed carbohydrates, and junk food may cause spikes in blood sugar, leading to hyperactivity, followed by energy crashes and irritability.

On the other hand, nutrient-dense meals help regulate blood sugar levels, providing steady energy and supporting cognitive function. Omega-3 fatty acids, for example, found in fish and flax seeds, are known to support brain health and improve concentration and mood. Similarly, foods rich in B vitamins help with energy metabolism and focus, while magnesium-rich foods, like leafy greens and nuts, are known to help calm the nervous system and improve sleep quality.

Studies have shown that children who eat a balanced diet rich in whole foods often perform better in school, show improved behavior, and have a more stable mood. Teaching kids about the relationship between what they eat and how they feel can also help them make healthier choices as they grow older.

Here are **10 healthy and kid-friendly ideas** for school lunches that pack nutrition while keeping things tasty and fun:

1. *Turkey & Avocado Wrap*

- **Ingredients**: Whole-grain wrap, sliced turkey, avocado, lettuce, and a little hummus.
- **Why It's Great**: Provides protein, healthy fats, and fiber to keep kids full and energized.

2. *Veggie-Packed Mini Muffins*

- **Ingredients**: Whole-wheat flour, shredded zucchini or carrots, a touch of honey, and a pinch of cinnamon.
- **Why It's Great**: These muffins sneak in veggies and can double as a snack. Perfect for kids who love bite-sized treats!

3. *Fruit & Yogurt Parfait*

- **Ingredients**: Greek yogurt, berries, sliced banana, and a sprinkle of granola.
- **Why It's Great**: This parfait is high in protein and probiotics, while also giving a natural boost of sweetness.

4. *Hummus & Veggie Sticks*

- **Ingredients**: Mini container of hummus, sliced carrots, cucumbers, and bell peppers.
- **Why It's Great**: Easy for dipping, this lunch adds fiber and healthy fats, and kids love the colorful variety.

5. Pita Pocket with Tuna Salad

- **Ingredients**: Whole-grain pita, tuna mixed with Greek yogurt, diced cucumber, and celery.
- **Why It's Great**: High in protein and omega-3, this is a tasty alternative to the usual sandwich.

6. DIY Pizza Roll-Ups

- **Ingredients**: Whole-grain tortilla, mozzarella cheese, turkey pepperoni, and marinara sauce for dipping.
- **Why It's Great**: Kids love this hands-on lunch, and it's a healthier twist on pizza.

7. Quinoa Salad with Veggies and Cheese

- **Ingredients**: Cooked quinoa, cherry tomatoes, cucumbers, diced cheese, and a light vinaigrette.
- **Why It's Great**: Packed with protein and fiber, this salad is refreshing and provides balanced nutrients.

8. Apple Slices with Nut Butter and Granola

- **Ingredients**: Sliced apple, almond or peanut butter, a sprinkle of granola.
- **Why It's Great**: This snack is crunchy, satisfying, and full of healthy fats and fiber to keep kids going.

9. Chicken & Cheese Quesadilla Slices

- **Ingredients**: Whole-wheat tortilla, shredded chicken, cheese, and a side of salsa.
- **Why It's Great**: Quesadilla slices are easy to eat and high in protein, with a side of salsa adding flavor and veggies.

10. Energy Balls

- **Ingredients**: Rolled oats, nut butter, honey, chia seeds, mini chocolate chips.
- **Why It's Great**: These bite-sized balls are fun, portable, and give a quick energy boost with natural sweetness and fiber.

These lunch ideas are packed with nutrition while offering variety and flavors that appeal to kids. Each option is designed to be easy to eat, flavorful, and filling for the school day!

Nutritional Benefits of Popular Diets

Each diet offers unique benefits and can suit different health goals and lifestyles. Here's an overview of the Mediterranean, keto, and carnivore diets, focusing on their potential advantages for balanced nutrition.

1. **Mediterranean Diet**

- **Overview:** The Mediterranean diet emphasizes plant-based foods, healthy fats (particularly olive oil), moderate protein, and whole grains. Inspired by the eating habits of countries around the Mediterranean Sea, this diet is celebrated for its heart-healthy benefits.

- **Nutritional Benefits:**
- Rich in Antioxidants: High consumption of fruits and vegetables provides essential vitamins, minerals, and antioxidants that support cellular health and reduce inflammation.
- Heart Health: Emphasis on monounsaturated fats (like olive oil) helps maintain healthy cholesterol levels and supports cardiovascular health.
- Balanced Macro nutrients: The diet balances complex carbs, protein, and healthy fats, supporting sustained energy and blood sugar regulation.

2. Keto Diet (Ketogenic)

- **Overview**: The keto diet is a high-fat, low-carbohydrate diet that aims to induce ketosis—a metabolic state where the body burns fat for fuel instead of carbohydrates.
- **Nutritional Benefits:**
- Supports Weight Management: Reduces appetite by stabilizing blood sugar levels and increasing satiety with healthy fats and moderate protein.
- Mental Clarity and Focus: Ketones, produced during ketosis, are a preferred fuel source for the brain and can enhance cognitive function.
- Reduced Inflammation: Low carb intake and higher fat consumption may help reduce inflammation markers, supporting overall health.

3. Carnivore Diet

- **Overview:** The carnivore diet is a highly restrictive diet that focuses on animal products exclusively. While highly debated, it emphasizes nutrient-dense meats, fish, and animal-based fats.

- **Nutritional Benefits**:
- Rich in High-Quality Protein: Provides complete proteins with all essential amino acids, supporting muscle growth, tissue repair, and immune health.
- Easy Digestion for Some: For those sensitive to plant-based foods, this diet may reduce digestive issues and symptoms.
- High in Bio available Nutrients: Animal products are dense in bio available iron, B vitamins, zinc, and omega-3 fatty acids, which are essential for many bodily functions.

Mediterranean Foods and Their Caloric Values

Below is a list of popular Mediterranean foods with approximate calorie counts per common serving sizes:

Food	Serving Size	Calories
Olive Oil	1 tbsp	120
Hummus	1/4 cup	100
Feta Cheese	1 oz	75
Salmon	3 oz (cooked)	180

Greek Yogurt
1 cup (plain)
100
Whole Wheat Pita
1 small (6-inch)
150
Chickpeas
1/2 cup (cooked)
120
Quinoa
1/2 cup (cooked)
110
Tomatoes
1 medium
25
Cucumbers
1/2 cup (sliced)
8
Spinach
1 cup (raw)
7
Bell Peppers
1 medium
25
Almonds
1 oz (about 23)
160
Olives
10 small
40
Lentils

1/2 cup (cooked)
115
Oranges
1 medium
62
Sardines
3 oz (canned)
140
Avocado
1/2 medium
120
Brown Rice
1/2 cup (cooked)
110
Eggplant
1 cup (cooked)
35

These calorie counts make it easier to plan balanced, portion-controlled meals within the Mediterranean framework, emphasizing nutrient-dense foods that support overall health.

Carey Reams and RBTI: The Role of pH Balance in Nutrient Absorption

Dr. Carey Reams, a pioneering biochemist and agricultural researcher, developed the Reams Biological Theory of Ionization (RBTI) as a method to understand and promote optimal health. At the core of RBTI is the concept that the body's pH balance is critical for nutrient absorption and overall wellness. According to Reams, a balanced pH not only optimizes bodily function but also determines how well nutrients are absorbed and utilized.

1. **The Ideal pH: 6.4**

- **Why 6.4?:** Carey Reams proposed that a body pH of 6.4 is ideal for nutrient absorption. This slightly acidic environment, he believed, allows the body to break down food efficiently, making it easier to absorb minerals and vitamins.
- **The Science Behind It:** When the body's pH is at 6.4, enzymes and digestive fluids function at their best, supporting processes like nutrient breakdown and assimilation. Reams found that when pH levels drift too high (alkaline) or too low (acidic), nutrient absorption decreases, leading to potential deficiencies and health imbalances.

2. **RBTI and pH Balance**

- **What is RBTI?:** Reams developed RBTI as a diagnostic tool to assess how well the body is processing nutrients. RBTI testing typically measures factors like sugar levels, nitrate levels, and pH balance to determine whether the body is functioning optimally.
- **Balancing pH:** According to RBTI principles, maintaining pH levels close to 6.4 can help prevent illnesses related to nutrient deficiencies. Reams believed that the body's organs, fluids, and cells work best when pH is balanced, which supports both physical and mental health.

3. **Practical Steps to Support pH Balance**

- **Diet and Nutrition:** Reams suggested that diet plays a primary role in maintaining pH. Eating a balance of vegetables, fruits, and lean proteins while minimizing processed foods can help stabilize pH levels around the 6.4 mark.

- **Hydration and Minerals:** Proper hydration, along with adequate minerals like calcium, potassium, and magnesium, also supports pH balance. Reams emphasized that minerals help regulate pH and prevent it from becoming too acidic or alkaline.

Why pH Matters for Your Family's Health

Understanding Reams' approach to pH can offer insight into your family's nutrition and wellness. By focusing on a balanced diet and monitoring pH levels, parents can support their children's ability to absorb and utilize nutrients more effectively, which is key to healthy growth and development.

A Personal Story of Healing Through Diet

I'll never forget when I was diagnosed with lupus. It was a difficult journey, filled with uncertainty and fatigue. After years of conventional treatments that left me feeling drained, I decided to explore alternative solutions. That's when I discovered the power of nutrition. I began shifting my diet, removing inflammatory foods (mainly sugar, wheat and oats along with other foods I found on an allergy test) and focusing on nutrient-dense meals that nourished my body. The results were nothing short of miraculous. My energy levels improved, my symptoms subsided, and I felt more in tune with my body than I had in years. The best part was my joint pain and chronic headaches and migraines disappeared. It was during this time that I truly learned that food is medicine—and it's a lesson I've carried with me ever since.

This personal experience reshaped my approach to health, and I've carried those lessons into my family's diet as well. It's not about perfection but about consistently making choices that support long-term wellness.

A Funny Anecdote on Kids and Healthy Eating

Kids have a way of reminding us about the simplicity of healthy eating. I remember a time when I was trying to prepare an elaborate "super food" meal, filled with ingredients I thought would impress my family—kale, quinoa, chia seeds, the whole nine yards. My son, unimpressed by my efforts, looked at the meal and asked, "Can't we just have apples and peanut butter?" At that moment, I realized that sometimes, simplicity is best. A sliced apple with a bit of nut butter offers fiber, healthy fats, and protein—everything he needs to fuel his little body without any fuss. Kids often remind us that healthy food doesn't have to be complicated. It's the simple, wholesome foods that often bring the most nourishment.

Food choices are crucial not only for physical health but also for behavior, emotional balance, and cognitive development in children. By embracing food as medicine, parents can take an active role in preventing illness and promoting long-term wellness. A diet filled with nutrient-dense whole foods serves as one of the most powerful tools for maintaining health and balance in our children's lives.

Embracing food as medicine is central to the crunchy lifestyle. It's about recognizing that the choices we make in the kitchen have a profound impact on our children's health and well-being. By focusing on whole, nutrient-rich foods, we give our kids the best possible foundation for physical, mental, and emotional growth.

In the next chapter, we'll examine another critical element of wellness: the environment in which our children grow. We'll explore the impact of air quality and how maintaining a clean, toxin-free environment can further support their health and development.

3

Breathing Life: The Importance of Clean Air

Have you ever stood by a mountain stream, taken a deep breath, and felt a sense of clarity and peace wash over you? That clean, crisp air feels different from the air we breathe in most city environments. It's lighter, fresher, and restorative. Clean air, especially in natural settings, can be transformative, not just for our sense of well-being, but for our overall health. Now imagine if the air your children breathe every day was as pure as that mountain air. Clean air is vital to their health and development, and in this chapter, we'll explore how understanding and managing air quality can have a profound effect on your child's wellness.

Clean air is foundational for health. From respiratory health to brain function, the quality of the air our children breathe plays a crucial role in their overall well-being. As parents, we can take proactive steps to ensure that the air inside and outside our homes is as clean as possible. Understanding air pollution and how to mitigate its effects is key to raising healthy, well-balanced children.

The Impact of Air Pollution on Child Health

We often take the air we breathe for granted. It's invisible, yet it impacts us daily, and its quality can vary dramatically depending on where we live and the environmental conditions around us. For children, who are still developing and tend to be more sensitive to environmental factors, air quality can have a profound impact on their health and overall well-being.

Types of Air Pollutants That Affect Children's Health

There are several types of pollutants commonly found in the air that can impact children's health, each affecting them in different ways.

1. **Particulate Matter (PM2.5 and PM10)**: Fine particles from sources like vehicle exhaust, industrial emissions, and wildfires can penetrate deep into the lungs.

- **Health Impact**: Linked to asthma, respiratory infections, reduced lung function, and even developmental delays.
- **Example**: A child exposed to high PM levels near highways may have a greater risk of respiratory issues compared to those living in less polluted areas.

1. **Ground-Level Ozone**: Often found in smog, ozone is formed when sunlight reacts with pollutants like car emissions and industrial chemicals.

- **Health Impact**: Causes airway inflammation, aggravates asthma, and can reduce lung growth in children.
- **Example**: Children in urban areas with high levels of ozone may experience more frequent asthma attacks on hot, sunny days when ozone levels are highest.

1. **Nitrogen Dioxide (NO2)**: Emitted from vehicles, power plants, and industrial facilities.

- **Health Impact**: Irritates the airways, contributes to asthma, and can reduce immunity to lung infections.
- **Example**: Children attending schools near busy roads or industrial zones may have higher NO2 exposure, increasing their likelihood of respiratory illnesses.

1. **Carbon Monoxide (CO)**: Produced by burning fossil fuels, CO interferes with oxygen delivery to organs.

- **Health Impact**: At high levels, it can cause headaches, dizziness, and even affect cognitive development.
- **Example**: Poorly ventilated indoor spaces with gas stoves or vehicles running in garages can pose a higher CO risk, especially for infants and young children.

1. **Volatile Organic Compounds (VOCs)**: Emitted from paints, cleaners, pesticides, and some building materials, VOCs can accumulate indoors.

- **Health Impact**: Linked to headaches, irritation, and potential long-term effects like neurodevelopmental issues.
- **Example**: In homes with high VOC-emitting products, children may experience increased irritability or concentration issues.

Health Effects of Air Pollution on Children

Children are particularly vulnerable to air pollution for several reasons:

- **Higher Respiratory Rate**: Children breathe faster than adults, taking in more air (and pollutants) relative to their body weight.
- **Developing Organs**: The lungs and brain are still developing, making them more susceptible to toxins.
- **Time Spent Outdoors**: Children often spend more time outside, increasing exposure, especially on days with poor air quality.

Examples of Health Issues Linked to Poor Air Quality in Children

1. **Asthma and Allergies**: Pollution, especially particulate matter and ozone, can trigger asthma attacks and exacerbate allergic reactions.

- **Example**: On days with high pollen and pollution levels, a child with asthma may experience severe symptoms or require additional medication.

1. **Developmental Delays and Learning Disabilities**: Studies have shown links between exposure to air pollutants (especially CO and heavy metals) and delays in cognitive and motor development.

- **Example**: Children living in highly industrialized areas have shown lower test scores and cognitive function compared to those in cleaner environments.

1. **Frequent Respiratory Infections**: Pollutants weaken children's immune responses, making them more susceptible to bronchitis, pneumonia, and other infections.

- **Example**: Children exposed to secondhand smoke or living near coal plants may experience more frequent colds and respiratory infections.

1. **Reduced Lung Growth**: Long-term exposure to air pollution can slow lung growth, which may impact a child's ability to be active and may lead to chronic respiratory

conditions later in life.

- **Example**: Children growing up in heavily polluted cities often exhibit slower lung growth than those in cleaner areas, affecting their endurance in physical activities.

Steps to Reduce Children's Exposure to Air Pollution

1. **Monitor Air Quality**: Use apps or websites that track daily air quality (e.g., AirVisual, AirNow). Limit outdoor play when pollution levels are high.

- **Tip**: Schedule outdoor activities for mornings or late afternoons when pollution tends to be lower, especially on high-traffic or hot days.

1. **Indoor Air Quality Improvements**: Use air purifiers with HEPA filters, avoid smoking indoors, and ventilate rooms frequently.

- **Tip**: Plants like spider plants, peace lilies, and snake plants can help improve indoor air quality by absorbing certain toxins.

1. **Create a "Clean Zone" in Bedrooms**: Make your child's bedroom a clean air zone by avoiding carpets (which can trap dust and pollutants), keeping windows closed on high-pollution days, and using non-toxic, VOC-free materials.

- **Tip**: Wash bedding and toys regularly to minimize allergens like dust mites.

1. **Use Natural Cleaning Products**: Opt for non-toxic, fragrance-free, and VOC-free cleaning supplies.

- **Tip**: Vinegar and baking soda are great natural alternatives to conventional cleaners and help keep indoor air cleaner.

1. **Limit Exposure to Traffic Pollution**: Try to walk or bike with your child along less busy routes and avoid standing near idling cars, as pollution is typically highest in close proximity to heavy traffic.

- **Tip**: When commuting, close car windows in heavy traffic and use the re-circulation mode on air conditioning to minimize outside air intake.

1. **Encourage a Nutritious Diet**: Antioxidant-rich foods (like berries, leafy greens, and nuts) can help counteract some of the harmful effects of pollution.

- **Tip**: Incorporate foods high in vitamins C and E, which help combat oxidative stress from pollutants.

1. **Reduce Dust and Allergens**: Vacuum with HEPA filters, and regularly clean floors and surfaces to minimize particulate buildup indoors.

- **Tip**: Use a damp cloth instead of a dry duster to avoid spreading dust into the air.

Air quality profoundly impacts children's health and development. By understanding the sources of air pollution and taking proactive steps to reduce exposure—both outdoors and inside the home—parents can help protect their children's health and promote long-term resilience against environmental stressors.

Respiratory Health and Development

Children's lungs are still developing well into their teenage years, making them especially vulnerable to the effects of air pollution. Exposure to pollutants like particulate matter (tiny particles suspended in the air), nitrogen dioxide, and ground-level ozone can have both immediate and long-term effects on respiratory health. For many children, especially those growing up in urban environments, air pollution can exacerbate asthma, bronchitis, and other respiratory conditions. It can also increase the risk of developing these conditions in children who are otherwise healthy.

Research has shown that children living in areas with high levels of air pollution are more likely to suffer from chronic respiratory problems and may experience reduced lung function as they grow older. Over time, this can lead to a higher risk of cardiovascular disease and other health complications.

But it's not just outdoor air pollution we need to worry about. Indoor air can sometimes be even more polluted than the air outside, due to factors like poor ventilation, household chemicals, and allergens. Long-term exposure to poor air quality can negatively affect cognitive development, immune function, and overall physical growth.

Improving Air Quality at Home

While we can't always control the air quality outside, there's a lot we can do to improve the air our children breathe at home. Creating a clean, well-ventilated living environment is one of the simplest yet most effective ways to protect your family's health.

Here are a few strategies for improving air quality in your home:

1. **Reduce Indoor Toxins:** Many common household products, such as cleaning supplies, air fresheners, and even furniture, can release harmful chemicals into the air. Opt for natural, non-toxic alternatives whenever possible. Look for cleaning products labeled "fragrance-free" and "non-toxic," and consider switching to natural cleaners like vinegar and baking soda.
2. **Improve Ventilation:** Ensure that your home is well-ventilated to allow fresh air to circulate. Open windows when weather permits, use exhaust fans in bathrooms and kitchens, and consider installing a high-efficiency particulate air (HEPA) filter to remove allergens and pollutants from the air.
3. **Houseplants:** Certain indoor plants, like spider plants, peace lilies, and snake plants, can help purify the air by removing toxins. They not only improve air quality but also bring a bit of nature indoors.
4. **Avoid Smoking Indoors:** Secondhand smoke is one of the most harmful indoor pollutants, especially for children. If anyone in your household smokes, ensure they do so outside and away from open windows and doors.
5. **Minimize the Use of Chemical Pesticides:** Pesticides and insecticides often contain toxic chemicals that can linger in the air and affect indoor air quality. Opt for natural alternatives or safe pest management practices.

Household Plants for Better Air Quality

Adding houseplants to your home is a simple, natural way to improve indoor air quality. Certain plants are particularly effective at filtering out common toxins, such as formaldehyde, benzene, and carbon monoxide. Here are some of the best plants for purifying the air:

1. Spider Plant (Chlorophytum comosum)

Benefits: Spider plants are easy to care for and highly effective at removing formaldehyde and xylene from the air. They're also non-toxic, making them safe for homes with pets.

Care: Place in indirect sunlight and water regularly.

2. Peace Lily (Spathiphyllum)

Benefits: Peace lilies help reduce levels of toxins like benzene, formaldehyde, and ammonia. They also increase indoor humidity, which can benefit respiratory health.

Care: Keep in a shady spot and water when the soil feels dry.

3. Snake Plant (Sansevieria trifasciata)

Benefits: Also known as "Mother-in-Law's Tongue," this plant is great at filtering out formaldehyde, benzene, and trichloroethylene. It also releases oxygen at night, making it ideal for bedrooms.

Care: Tolerates low light and needs very little water.

4. Aloe Vera (Aloe barbadensis miller)

Benefits: Aloe vera not only filters the air but also has healing properties for minor burns and skin irritations. It helps remove formaldehyde and benzene, which are often found in household cleaners.

Care: Place in bright, indirect sunlight and water sparingly.

5. Boston Fern (Nephrolepis exaltata)

Benefits: Boston ferns are natural humidifiers and excellent at removing pollutants such as formaldehyde and xylene.

Care: They thrive in humid environments, so mist them regularly and keep the soil moist.

6. Rubber Plant (Ficus elastica)

Benefits: Rubber plants are particularly good at removing formaldehyde from the air. Their large, waxy leaves absorb pollutants and convert them into nutrients.

Care: Place in medium to bright light and water when the soil dries out.

7. Bamboo Palm (Chamaedorea seifrizii)

Benefits: This palm is a powerful air purifier, removing formaldehyde, benzene, and trichloroethylene. It also adds moisture to the air, making it great for dry environments.

Care: Thrives in indirect light and needs regular watering.

8. English Ivy (Hedera helix)

Benefits: English ivy is effective at reducing airborne mold and formaldehyde levels. It's particularly useful in bathrooms and other humid areas.

Care: Requires moderate sunlight and regular watering.

9. Pothos (Epipremnum aureum)

Benefits: Pothos is one of the easiest plants to grow and helps filter out formaldehyde, benzene, and carbon monoxide.

Care: Grows in low light and only needs occasional watering.

10. Gerbera Daisy (Gerbera jamesonii)

Benefits: These vibrant flowers are great at removing benzene and formaldehyde and can also improve indoor air quality by absorbing carbon dioxide and releasing oxygen at night.

Care: Needs bright light and regular watering.

Green Your Space for Clean Air

Houseplants not only beautify your home but also improve air quality by filtering out harmful toxins. Adding any of these air-purifying plants to your home can help create a healthier living environment for you and your family.

Protecting Your Family from EMF and Frequency Exposure

In today's digital world, we are constantly surrounded by electromagnetic fields (EMFs) from devices like smartphones, WI-Fi routers, and electronic appliances. While these technologies are essential for modern living, there is growing concern about the potential health risks associated with long-term EMF exposure, particularly for children whose developing bodies and brains may be more sensitive to these frequencies.

EMFs are invisible waves of energy, also known as electromagnetic radiation, which are emitted by electrical and wireless devices. These fields can interfere with the body's natural frequencies and potentially contribute to issues like sleep disturbances, headaches, fatigue, and increased stress.

Understanding the Risks of EMF Exposure

While research is ongoing, several studies have highlighted possible connections between EMF exposure and health problems. Some of the concerns include:

- **Sleep Disruptions**: EMFs can interfere with the body's production of melatonin, the hormone responsible for regulating sleep. Children who are exposed to high levels of EMF radiation may have trouble falling or staying asleep.
- **Cognitive and Behavioral Effects**: Prolonged exposure

to high levels of EMFs may affect brain development in children, potentially leading to issues with focus, attention, and mood regulation.

- **Increased Stress and Fatigue**: EMFs have been linked to increased oxidative stress, which can contribute to chronic fatigue and weakened immunity over time.

How to Reduce EMF Exposure for Your Family

While it's impossible to completely eliminate EMF exposure in our modern world, there are several ways to minimize it and protect your family's health:

1. **Create an EMF-Free Sleep Environment**:

- Remove electronic devices from bedrooms, especially children's rooms. Try to keep phones, tablets, and WI-Fi routers out of the bedroom at night.
- Use an analog alarm clock instead of a digital one to minimize exposure while sleeping.
- Consider turning off WI-Fi routers at night or placing them as far away from living and sleeping spaces as possible.

1. **Limit Screen Time and Device Use**:

- Encourage children to take regular breaks from screens, and use devices in "airplane mode" when possible to reduce radiation exposure.
- Use wired internet connections rather than relying on WI-Fi whenever possible, especially for long periods of use like streaming or gaming.

1. **EMF Protection Devices and Clothing**:

- EMF-blocking devices, such as shields and cases for phones, tablets, and laptops, can reduce direct exposure. Look for products made from conductive materials like silver that block radiation.
- You can also find EMF-protective clothing, such as hats and blankets, made from shielding fabrics that can offer extra protection, especially for babies and young children.

1. **Create Distance from Devices**:

- Keeping a reasonable distance from electronics can significantly reduce EMF exposure. Encourage children not to hold tablets or phones directly against their bodies for extended periods, and use speakerphone or wired headphones when making calls.
- Maintain distance from household appliances like microwaves or televisions while they are in use.

1. **Grounding (Earthing)**:

- Grounding, or walking barefoot on natural surfaces like grass, sand, or soil, helps discharge built-up electrical energy in the body. Regular grounding has been shown to reduce stress, improve sleep, and help neutralize the effects of EMF exposure.

1. **Use EMF Meters**:

- EMF meters are tools that can measure electromagnetic

radiation in your home, allowing you to identify areas with high EMF levels. This can help you better understand where to make changes or limit time spent in certain areas of your home.

The Importance of Frequency Balance

Our bodies operate on their own natural frequencies, and exposure to artificial EMFs can disrupt that balance. In holistic health, maintaining energetic balance is critical for physical and emotional well-being. Tools such as biofeedback or energy medicine can help identify areas where the body's frequencies are out of alignment and offer corrective strategies, such as energy healing or frequency-specific therapies.

Biofeedback and Frequency Protection:

- Biofeedback technology can help monitor and balance your body's physiological responses, especially after prolonged EMF exposure. It's an excellent tool for identifying stress caused by environmental factors, and it can support relaxation and healing.
- Energy healing techniques such as Reiki or frequency-specific micro-current therapy can also be helpful in restoring the body's natural energetic balance after frequent EMF exposure.

Protecting Your Family from EMFs for Better Health

While we can't completely avoid EMF exposure, we can take proactive steps to limit it in our homes and protect our children's developing brains and bodies. By creating EMF-free zones, limiting screen time, using protective devices, and encouraging grounding activities, you can reduce the impact of electromagnetic radiation on your family's health. Maintaining a balanced frequency through holistic practices such as biofeedback and energy healing can also help mitigate the effects of modern technology on well-being.

Grounding: Reconnecting with the Earth for Better Health

In our modern, technology-driven world, many of us have become disconnected from the earth. Grounding, also known as earthing, is a practice that involves making direct physical contact with the earth's surface, such as walking barefoot on grass, soil, sand, or even water. This simple act allows us to reconnect with the earth's natural energy, which can have a range of health benefits for both adults and children.

What is Grounding?

Grounding is based on the idea that the earth carries a subtle electric charge that can help balance and stabilize our own body's energy. Our ancestors were naturally grounded because they lived closer to nature and spent most of their time outdoors. Today, many of us are constantly insulated from the earth by shoes, buildings, and other man-made surfaces, which limits our exposure to this natural energy source.

By making direct contact with the earth, we allow our bodies to absorb the earth's electrons, which may help neutralize free radicals and restore balance to our body's energy systems.

The Benefits of Grounding

- **Reduced Inflammation**: Studies suggest that grounding can reduce inflammation in the body, which is often linked to chronic health conditions.

- **Improved Sleep**: Many people report better sleep quality after grounding regularly. Grounding may help balance cortisol levels, which can lead to a deeper, more restful sleep.
- **Stress Relief**: Grounding can help lower stress by calming the nervous system. It has been shown to reduce feelings of anxiety and improve mood.
- **Better Circulation**: Physical contact with the earth can improve blood flow, which supports heart health and overall circulation.
- **Boosted Immunity**: Grounding may help strengthen the immune system by supporting the body's ability to fight off infections and heal more quickly.

How to Practice Grounding

Grounding is simple, and it doesn't require any special equipment. Here are some easy ways you and your kids can practice grounding in everyday life:

1. **Walk Barefoot Outside**: The easiest way to ground is to walk barefoot on grass, soil, sand, or any natural surface. Make this a fun activity with your kids by exploring parks, beaches, or even your own backyard.
2. **Lie on the Ground**: Encourage your children to lie down on the grass and feel the earth beneath them. This is a great way to relax and connect with nature during outdoor play.
3. **Garden Barefoot**: If you enjoy gardening, try doing it without shoes. Working with the soil and being barefoot at the same time doubles the grounding effect.
4. **Use Grounding Mats or Sheets**: If going outside isn't always an option, grounding mats and sheets are available. These products are designed to mimic the effect of walking

barefoot by connecting you to the earth's natural energy, even indoors.

5. **Spend Time in Nature**: Simply spending time in natural environments, such as hiking, swimming in a natural body of water, or sitting under a tree, helps your body absorb the benefits of the earth's energy.

Grounding is a simple yet powerful practice that reconnects us with the earth's natural energy, offering a range of physical and emotional benefits. By encouraging your children to spend more time outdoors and practice grounding, you're supporting their overall health and helping them establish a deep connection with nature from an early age.

A Family's Experience: Moving from Urban to Rural Living

The Jones family lived in a bustling city for years, but as their children began to develop frequent respiratory issues, they started to wonder if their urban environment was contributing to the problem. After years of dealing with chronic coughs and asthma flare-ups, they made the difficult decision to move to a rural area, where the air was cleaner and nature was more accessible. The change was remarkable. Within months of moving, the children's symptoms significantly improved. They no longer needed daily asthma medication, and their energy levels increased. The family quickly realized how much of an impact clean air had on their overall health. It was a transformative experience that reinforced the importance of their environment on their children's well-being.

Community Efforts to Combat Pollution

In a small town in the Midwest, a group of mothers banded together to address rising pollution levels in their area. Their children had been experiencing a surge in respiratory issues, which they suspected was linked to a nearby industrial plant. The moms organized a grassroots movement, raising awareness in their community about the dangers of air pollution and petitioning local government officials to enforce stricter environmental regulations. Their efforts paid off—within a few years, the plant was required to reduce its emissions, and air quality in the area improved dramatically. The mothers' commitment to protecting their children's health serves as a powerful reminder of the impact that community activism can have in safeguarding the environment.

Every breath matters. Maintaining good air quality, both inside and outside the home, is an essential part of holistic health practices for children. By paying attention to the environment our children live and play in, we can help protect their developing lungs, support their immune systems, and ensure that they grow up in a healthy, nurturing environment.

This chapter highlights how nurturing environments, like clean air, contribute to balanced child development. By taking proactive steps to reduce exposure to harmful pollutants, both indoors and outdoors, we can create healthier spaces for our children to thrive.

In the next chapter, we'll explore a highly debated topic in the world of health and parenting: the impact of vaccinations on child health. We'll take a closer look at the various perspectives and considerations parents face when making decisions about vaccinations.

4

A Different View on Vaccinations

Few topics in parenting ignite as much debate as vaccinations. It's a discussion that's often heated and divided, with strong opinions on both sides. Whether you choose to vaccinate or explore alternative options, the decisions we make as parents shape our children's health in profound ways. For many parents, the vaccination debate is not just theoretical—it's personal. In this chapter, we explore an alternative perspective on vaccinations through the lens of parents who have faced these choices firsthand. Here's the story of one mother whose experience shifted her approach to health and wellness, offering insight into the complexities surrounding vaccines.

Vaccinations have been a cornerstone of public health for decades, but for some parents, concerns about their long-term impact on child health have led them to seek alternative paths. This chapter examines the history and evolution of vaccinations, as well as the critical importance of informed choice in parenting. We will explore case studies from both sides of the debate, encouraging parents to make health decisions based on personal experiences and broader health considerations.

History and Evolution of Vaccinations

Vaccinations have saved millions of lives since their widespread introduction in the 20th century. Diseases that once devastated populations, such as smallpox, polio, and measles, have been largely controlled or eradicated thanks to global vaccination efforts. However, as vaccine programs expanded, so did questions about their safety, particularly in relation to potential side effects and long-term health outcomes.

In the early years of vaccination, there was little room for debate—vaccines were seen as miracle solutions to deadly diseases. But over time, as more vaccines were developed and administered at younger ages, some parents began to question whether the benefits always outweigh the risks. Concerns about vaccine ingredients, the sheer number of vaccines on the childhood schedule, and potential links to conditions like autism fueled a growing movement of parents seeking more control over their children's health care decisions.

Today, while the medical community overwhelmingly supports vaccines, there are parents who advocate for a more cautious approach. For these parents, the decision to vaccinate (or not) is deeply personal, influenced by their family's health history, their children's unique needs, and their own research into alternative health practices.

Case Studies on Vaccination Outcomes

Balanced insights into the vaccination debate require looking at the outcomes from both sides. For many families, vaccines have provided critical protection against diseases, with little to no adverse effects. On the other hand, some families report experiences of adverse reactions that have led them to question the safety of vaccines. Let's explore both perspectives.

- **Pro-Vaccine Perspective:** For parents who follow the standard vaccination schedule, the benefits often far outweigh the risks. Their children are protected against potentially deadly diseases, and side effects, if any, are usually mild and temporary. Many parents feel confident in their choice, reassured by decades of research supporting the safety and efficacy of vaccines. These families often emphasize the importance of herd immunity, where vaccinated individuals help protect those who are unable to get vaccinated due to medical reasons.
- **Alternative Perspective:** On the other hand, there are families who have had different experiences. Some report that their children experienced adverse reactions after vaccinations—ranging from high fevers and seizures to developmental regressions that raised concerns about long-term health effects. While these cases are rare, they have prompted some parents to delay or skip certain vaccines, or to explore alternative vaccine schedules that spread out the doses over a longer period of time.

Both perspectives highlight the complexity of the vaccination debate. It's not a one-size-fits-all decision, and each family's experience is unique.

Informed Choice in Parenting

Making informed health decisions is a cornerstone of the crunchy lifestyle. Whether it's choosing natural remedies or considering alternative health practices, informed choice empowers parents to do what they believe is best for their children. The same holds true for vaccines. Vaccination is a deeply personal decision, and parents must weigh the benefits and risks in the context of their own family's health history and values.

An informed choice means doing your own research, consulting with medical professionals you trust, and considering your child's individual needs. It also means understanding the broader implications of your decision—both for your child and for the community. For some parents, this may mean following the standard vaccination schedule; for others, it may mean seeking alternatives or delaying certain vaccines.

In-Depth Evolution of the Childhood Vaccine Schedule

1980s: The Foundation

In the 1980s, the childhood vaccine schedule was simpler, covering a few essential vaccines to protect against some of the most dangerous diseases:

- **DTP (Diphtheria, Tetanus, Pertussis)**: A combined vaccine given to protect against three serious bacterial diseases.
- **Polio (OPV/IPV)**: Oral polio vaccine was standard, later replaced by the inactivated polio vaccine to avoid the rare risk of vaccine-derived polio.
- **MMR (Measles, Mumps, Rubella)**: Introduced in the 1970s, this vaccine targeted three viral infections that could cause severe health complications.

Rationale for Changes: The 1980s schedule focused on diseases that caused high mortality or severe complications. However, concerns about vaccine-related side effects and an increase in cases of vaccine-preventable diseases led to an expansion of the schedule to cover more diseases.

Early 1990s: Hepatitis B and Hib Introduction

Two new vaccines were added to the schedule, expanding coverage:

- **Hepatitis B (1991)**: Initially targeted at high-risk populations (e.g., healthcare workers), the CDC expanded it to all newborns by 1991 due to rising cases of chronic hepatitis B infections in children, often transmitted at birth or early childhood.
- **Hib (Haemophilus influenzae type b) (1990)**: Added to prevent bacterial infections that could lead to meningitis, pneumonia, and epiglottitis in young children. This vaccine greatly reduced Hib-related illnesses.

Why These Vaccines Were Added: Both vaccines targeted diseases spread through blood or respiratory droplets, reducing the risk of severe complications and chronic health issues in early childhood.

Mid-1990s: Chickenpox Vaccine

- **Varicella (Chickenpox) (1995)**: Introduced to prevent chickenpox, a common childhood illness that could lead to complications like bacterial infections and pneumonia. Initially a single dose, it was expanded to a two-dose series in 2006 due to breakthrough infections.

Rationale: Although chickenpox is often mild, the vaccine reduced hospitalizations and complications from severe cases. It also reduced economic impacts by preventing parents from missing work to care for sick children.

Late 1990s to Early 2000s: Rota-virus, Pneumococcal, and Hepatitis A

Three vaccines were introduced between 1998 and 2000 to address viral and bacterial diseases that cause significant morbidity:

- **Rota-virus (1998, reintroduced 2006)**: A vaccine to prevent severe diarrhea and dehydration in infants and young children. Initially introduced in 1998, it was withdrawn due to safety concerns and reintroduced in 2006 with a safer formulation.
- **PCV7 (Pneumococcal Conjugate) (2000)**: This vaccine protected against seven strains of Streptococcus pneumoniae, which can cause meningitis, sepsis, and pneumonia.
- **Hepatitis A (1996, routine recommendation in 2006)**: Initially targeted at high-risk areas, it was added to the standard schedule to prevent hepatitis A virus infections, often spread through contaminated food and water.

Reasoning: These vaccines addressed diseases with high hospitalization rates among young children. The pneumococcal vaccine, in particular, significantly reduced severe respiratory infections and meningitis cases in infants and toddlers.

2006–2010: HPV, Meningococcal, and Expanded Pneumococcal Coverage

The schedule expanded again with vaccines that targeted specific populations and age groups:

- **HPV (Human Papillomavirus) (2006)**: First introduced for girls at ages 11-12 to prevent cervical and other HPV-related cancers. It was later expanded to boys and included more strains to broaden protection.
- **Meningococcal (MCV4) (2005)**: Introduced for adolescents,

targeting meningitis caused by meningococcal bacteria. The CDC recommends it for preteens and teens, particularly in communal living settings like dorms.

- **PCV13 (2010)**: This updated pneumococcal vaccine replaced PCV7 and covered 13 strains of Streptococcus pneumoniae, further reducing invasive pneumococcal disease rates.

Rationale for Expansion: These additions reflected advancements in targeting cancers and infections affecting adolescents. The HPV vaccine was especially noteworthy for its potential to prevent specific cancers, aligning with public health goals to reduce HPV-related cancer rates over time.

2010s to Present: Refinements and Seasonal Recommendations

The schedule has continued to adapt based on new data and changing health needs:

- **Annual Influenza Vaccine**: While flu shots have been available for decades, they became a routine recommendation for children starting at 6 months to prevent seasonal flu and related complications.
- **Meningococcal B (MenB) (2014)**: Added for specific high-risk groups or during outbreaks, as MenB only covers certain strains of meningococcal disease not included in MCV4.

Current Trends: The focus has shifted toward refining existing vaccines (e.g., updated influenza strains annually) and increasing coverage in response to outbreaks or emerging strains, such as MenB.

Summary of Key Vaccine Additions by Decade

Decade
Vaccines Added
Purpose

1980s
DTP, Polio, MMR
Foundation of the schedule, focusing on high-risk diseases
1990s
Hepatitis B, Hib, Varicella
Expanded coverage, preventable infections
Early 2000s
PCV7, Rotavirus, Hepatitis A
Reduced respiratory and gastrointestinal infections
Mid-2000 to 2009
HPV, Meningococcal (MCV4)
Cancer prevention, targeted adolescent vaccines
2010s
PCV13, Influenza, MenB
Broadened protection, adapted to emerging strains

Key Vaccine-Related Cases

Historically, several landmark cases have shaped vaccine policy and public understanding of vaccine safety and efficacy. These cases illustrate the complexities of balancing public health needs with individual rights and concerns, especially where children are involved.

1. **Jacobson v. Massachusetts (1905)**

- **Overview**: This Supreme Court case addressed the consti-

tutionality of mandatory smallpox vaccination during an outbreak in Cambridge, Massachusetts.
- **Ruling**: The court upheld the authority of states to enforce mandatory vaccination laws, stating that individual freedoms can be limited to protect public health.
- **Impact**: Jacobson v. Massachusetts set a precedent that states could mandate vaccines for the greater good, forming the foundation for modern school immunization requirements.

2. Bruesewitz v. Wyeth LLC (2011)

- **Overview**: This case involved a claim under the National Childhood Vaccine Injury Act (NCVIA), which provides compensation for vaccine injuries but also limits lawsuits against vaccine manufacturers.
- **Ruling**: The Supreme Court ruled that vaccine manufacturers are not liable for vaccine injuries if the vaccine is "properly prepared and accompanied by proper directions and warnings."
- **Impact**: This ruling reinforced the protection for vaccine manufacturers under the NCVIA, aiming to stabilize vaccine availability and public confidence while ensuring an avenue for compensation in rare cases of injury.

3. Hannah Poling Case (2008)

- **Overview**: In 2008, the family of Hannah Poling, a child who developed autism-like symptoms after receiving multiple vaccines, was awarded compensation through the Vaccine Injury Compensation Program (VICP).

- **Significance**: The government did not link vaccines to autism but acknowledged that the vaccines "aggravated" an underlying mitochondrial disorder in Poling, leading to her symptoms.
- **Impact**: Although not a conclusive case of vaccine-induced autism, this case sparked considerable public debate and contributed to increased vaccine hesitancy, especially among parents of children with underlying health concerns.

4. Doe v. Bolton and Vaccine Exemptions

- **Overview**: Although this case did not specifically address vaccines, it set a precedent for medical exemptions under constitutional law.
- **Significance**: The decision supported the right to medical exemptions, paving the way for later state legislation that permits medical and, in some cases, religious or philosophical exemptions to vaccination requirements.
- **Impact**: States have interpreted this ruling in various ways, leading to diverse exemption policies across the U.S., with some states narrowing and others expanding allowable exemptions.

5. Wakefield and MMR-Autism Controversy (1998)

- **Overview**: Dr. Andrew Wakefield published a study in 1998 suggesting a link between the MMR (measles, mumps, rubella) vaccine and autism. This study was later retracted, and Wakefield's medical license was revoked due to unethical research practices.
- **Outcome**: Subsequent studies found no link between the

MMR vaccine and autism, and the controversy is now regarded as one of the most significant cases of medical misinformation in modern history.

- **Impact**: Wakefield's study contributed to lasting vaccine hesitancy, particularly around MMR, and led to increased research into vaccine safety to restore public trust.

6. National Vaccine Injury Compensation Program (VICP) (1986)

- **Overview**: The VICP was established in response to lawsuits claiming injuries from the DTP (diphtheria, tetanus, pertussis) vaccine, which threatened vaccine supply due to rising costs.
- **Significance**: The program provides compensation for proven vaccine injuries while protecting manufacturers from direct lawsuits, aiming to keep vaccines accessible and affordable.
- **Impact**: VICP has compensated thousands of claims while helping maintain vaccine supply and public trust by addressing rare adverse reactions.

7. Zucht v. King (1922)

- **Overview**: This case upheld a Texas ordinance that required children to be vaccinated against smallpox before attending public school.
- **Ruling**: The Supreme Court ruled that states have the authority to mandate vaccinations as a condition for school attendance.
- **Impact**: This ruling reinforced the right of states to require

vaccinations for school entry, a policy still in effect and foundational to today's public health policies.

These cases underscore the complexity of vaccine policy, balancing individual freedoms with public health imperatives. While Jacobson v. Massachusetts established the basis for mandatory vaccines, subsequent cases have refined the balance between accessibility, safety, and liability. They highlight the need for robust public health protections and the importance of informed decision-making for parents navigating vaccination choices.

A Mother's Experience: Autism Diagnosis After MMR Vaccine

One mother, Jessica, vividly recalls the moment when her life changed. Her first child, Adam, had been a healthy and active toddler, hitting all of his developmental milestones on time. But shortly after receiving the MMR (measles, mumps, and rubella) vaccine, she noticed a change. Adam stopped making eye contact, became less communicative, and eventually lost the ability to speak. After months of evaluations, Adam was diagnosed with autism.

Jessica began to research alternative perspectives on vaccinations, seeking answers that the medical community couldn't provide. While there is no conclusive evidence linking vaccines to autism, Jessica's personal experience led her to make a different choice with her second child. For her daughter, she chose an alternative vaccination schedule, delaying certain vaccines and using natural immune support to mitigate any potential risks. She emphasizes that this decision was based on her family's unique circumstances and that every parent must make the best decision for their own children.

Diverse Family Accounts on Vaccination Choices

Many families have shared their experiences on both sides of the vaccination debate, highlighting how personal and varied the journey can be.

- **For Vaccination:** The Smith family chose to follow the full vaccination schedule for their children. They believed that the risks of vaccine-preventable diseases far outweighed the risks of side effects. For them, the decision was about protecting not only their own kids but also the broader community. Their children experienced only mild reactions to vaccines, such as a low-grade fever, and they felt confident in their choice.
- **Against Vaccination:** The Jones family, on the other hand, chose to skip several vaccines after their eldest child had a severe reaction to the DTaP vaccine. They felt that the medical community didn't take their concerns seriously, so they sought out a holistic pediatrician who supported their decision to use natural remedies and immune support in place of certain vaccines.

These diverse accounts reflect the complexity of the vaccination decision. Whether parents choose to vaccinate or not, what's important is that the decision is made with careful consideration and a deep understanding of the implications.

Guide to Politely Declining a Vaccine

Deciding whether or not to vaccinate your child is a deeply personal choice. If you choose to decline a vaccine, it's important to approach the conversation with your healthcare provider in a respectful and informed way. Here are steps you can take to politely and confidently express your decision:

Step 1: Be Informed and Prepared

Before your appointment, research the vaccine being offered. Understand the benefits, risks, and any potential alternatives. This allows you to have an informed discussion with your healthcare provider and shows that your decision is based on thoughtful consideration rather than fear or misinformation.

Step 2: Use Clear and Respectful Language

When you're ready to decline a vaccine, it's important to remain calm, polite, and clear in your communication. Here's an example of how to phrase your decision respectfully:

- *"Thank you for the information. After researching and considering our options, we've decided to decline this vaccine for now."*

Step 3: Express Appreciation for Their Expertise

Acknowledging the healthcare provider's role and expertise shows that you respect their perspective, even if you don't agree with their recommendation. This can help keep the conversation respectful and open.

- *"I appreciate your concern and understand the benefits from a medical perspective, but we feel this is the best decision for our family right now."*

Step 4: Ask for Alternative Suggestions

If the vaccine was suggested to prevent a specific illness, ask if there are any natural or alternative ways to boost immunity. This opens the conversation for a more holistic approach to health.

- *"Are there any natural ways we can support my child's immune system instead?"*

Step 5: Reaffirm Your Decision Gently

If the provider pushes back or tries to persuade you, stay calm and reaffirm your decision without engaging in a debate. Keeping the tone firm but respectful will show that you are confident in your choice.

- *"I understand your concerns, but we've done our research and feel comfortable with our decision to decline this vaccine."*

Step 6: Know Your Rights

If you're asked to sign a waiver or document acknowledging that you are declining the vaccine, ask for clarification and ensure you fully understand what you're signing. It's your right to ask questions and make sure the documentation aligns with your decision.

Sample Conversations for Common Scenarios

If the provider says: "This vaccine is very important for preventing serious illness."

You can say:

- *"I understand that, and we've taken the time to research the risks and benefits. At this time, we've decided to take a more natural approach to support our child's health."*

If the provider says: "It's recommended by all major health organizations."

You can say:

- *"I know there's a lot of support for this vaccine, but after reviewing all of the information and considering our family's unique needs, we feel this is the right choice for us."*

If the provider says: "Are you sure? It's a safe vaccine."

You can say:

- *"We've taken the time to look at the safety data, and we're comfortable with our decision. Thank you for your concern."*

Respectful Decision-Making

By approaching the conversation with respect and confidence, you can assert your decision to decline a vaccine in a way that maintains a positive relationship with your healthcare provider. Remember that you have the right to make decisions about your child's health, and you can do so in a way that is informed, polite, and assertive.

Navigating Vaccine Exemptions for School and Daycare

In most countries and U.S. states, children are required to have certain vaccinations to attend school or daycare. However, many parents choose to delay, space out, or decline vaccinations for personal, religious, or medical reasons. If you've made the decision to avoid or selectively vaccinate your child, there are legal options available to help you navigate school and daycare requirements.

Here's how to understand the laws and assert your right to make health decisions for your child.

1. Know Your Legal Rights

Vaccine exemption laws vary by country and state, but in many places, parents have the legal right to opt out of vaccines required for school and daycare attendance under specific conditions.

In the United States, there are three main types of vaccine exemptions:

- **Medical Exemptions**: These exemptions are granted when a licensed healthcare provider certifies that a child cannot receive certain vaccines due to medical reasons, such as allergies, compromised immunity, or a history of adverse reactions. Medical exemptions must typically be renewed annually and must be signed by a doctor.
- **Religious Exemptions**: In some states, parents can opt out of vaccinating their children based on their religious beliefs. No specific religion needs to be cited, but you must submit a formal statement to the school outlining your religious opposition to vaccines. Some states may require you to explain how your beliefs conflict with vaccinations.
- **Philosophical Exemptions**: These exemptions allow parents to decline vaccines for personal or philosophical reasons. These are sometimes referred to as "conscientious objector" exemptions. Philosophical exemptions are only available in certain states.

Important: As of 2024, the availability of religious and philosophical exemptions is restricted or eliminated in some states due to changes in state laws. Always check the specific laws in your state or country to understand which exemptions are available to you.

2. Understanding Vaccine Exemption Laws by State

Vaccine laws are different depending on where you live. Here's a brief overview of how exemptions work in the U.S.:

- **States That Allow Medical, Religious, and Philosophical Exemptions**: Some states allow all three types of exemptions. For example, Idaho, Utah, and Texas provide families with options for opting out based on personal or religious beliefs as well as for medical reasons.
- **States That Only Allow Medical and Religious Exemptions**: States like Florida, Pennsylvania, and Ohio allow both medical and religious exemptions but do not accept philosophical exemptions.
- **States That Only Allow Medical Exemptions**: A few states, such as California, New York, and Maine, have removed religious and philosophical exemptions, allowing only medical exemptions. These states have more stringent vaccination laws, but parents can still apply for medical exemptions if appropriate.

To check the laws in your state, visit your state's Department of Health website or consult the National Vaccine Information Center (NVIC), which provides updated information on vaccine laws and exemptions.

3. How to File for a Vaccine Exemption

Once you know the type of exemption available in your state, follow these steps to file for an exemption:

1. **Request an Exemption Form**: Contact your child's school or daycare and request the necessary exemption forms. Some states offer the forms online through their health department websites, while others require you to submit a written statement.
2. **Complete the Paperwork**: Fill out the exemption form completely, specifying the reason for your exemption (medical, religious, or philosophical). If it's a medical exemption, you will need a doctor's signature.
3. **Submit the Form**: Return the completed exemption form to your child's school or daycare. Some states require you to renew your exemption yearly, so check if your state has an annual requirement.
4. **Be Prepared for Follow-Up**: In states where exemptions are allowed, schools or daycare centers may follow up with you to ensure compliance with state laws. Some schools may ask for additional documentation or information, particularly if it's a medical exemption.

4. Communicating with Schools and Daycare Providers

When discussing your decision with schools or daycare providers, it's important to approach the conversation calmly and respectfully. Here are a few tips:

- **Be Confident and Informed**: Know the exemption laws in your state and be prepared to explain your rights. Bring copies of the relevant state laws or exemption forms if needed.
- **Stay Respectful**: Keep in mind that school administrators

are often just following the policies required by the state. Stay calm and respectful during the conversation, even if they have questions or concerns about your exemption.

- **Focus on Your Child's Health**: Emphasize that you are making the best decision for your child's health based on research and careful consideration. If it's a medical exemption, highlight your child's specific needs.

5. Legal Protections for Vaccine Choice

Several legal frameworks in the U.S. protect the rights of parents to make health decisions for their children:

- **Parental Rights Doctrine**: This principle, established by the U.S. Supreme Court, affirms that parents have the fundamental right to direct the upbringing and care of their children, including making healthcare decisions such as vaccination.
- **First Amendment Rights**: Religious exemptions are protected under the First Amendment, which guarantees the right to freedom of religion. If your state offers religious exemptions, you can exercise your constitutional right to decline vaccines based on your religious beliefs.
- **National Vaccine Injury Compensation Program (VICP)**: This federal program recognizes that vaccines can cause injury and provides compensation for those affected. It's a reminder that vaccines carry risks, and parents have the right to assess those risks and make informed choices.

6. Building a Support Network

Navigating the vaccine exemption process can be challenging, but you don't have to do it alone. Join support groups and connect with like-minded parents who are navigating similar challenges. Online communities and local groups focused on holistic parenting or vaccine choice can provide resources, advice, and encouragement.

Some resources for support and information include:

- **National Vaccine Information Center (NVIC)**
- **Children's Health Defense**
- **Holistic Moms Network**

These organizations provide helpful tools and legal resources for navigating exemption laws and asserting your right to make informed health decisions for your child.

Safe Alternatives for Vaccines

While vaccines are a well-known preventive measure, some parents seek alternative ways to support their child's immune system naturally. Alternatives to vaccination are not widely supported by mainstream medical communities as substitutes for traditional immunization but may be used by families as complementary approaches to health. It's important to consult with a healthcare professional before pursuing alternative routes, especially for children.

1. Strengthening Immunity Naturally

Boosting the immune system is foundational in holistic health. A strong immune system is a natural defense against many infections, and certain lifestyle practices can promote immune resilience.

- **Balanced Nutrition**: A nutrient-dense diet rich in antioxidants (e.g., vitamins C and E), minerals like zinc, and whole foods strengthens immunity. Foods like leafy greens, berries, nuts, and lean proteins are excellent for immune health.

- **Probiotics**: Healthy gut flora is crucial for immune function. Probiotics from sources like yogurt, kefir, sauerkraut, and probiotic supplements support gut health and help reduce infection risks.
- **Daily Exercise and Sleep**: Physical activity and adequate sleep are vital for maintaining a healthy immune system, especially in children. Aim for 8–10 hours of sleep for young children and regular outdoor play.

2. Homeopathic Nosodes

Homeopathic nosodes are diluted preparations made from diseased tissue or other pathogen sources. They're sometimes used as an alternative to vaccination, although their effectiveness and safety as a vaccine substitute remain controversial in traditional medical fields.

- **What are Nosodes?** Nosodes are created by taking the original substance (e.g., bacteria or virus material), diluting it multiple times, and preparing it according to homeopathic principles. They aim to stimulate the body's immune response without introducing a live pathogen.
- **Commonly Used Nosodes**: Nosodes exist for various diseases, including whooping cough, measles, and influenza. They are typically administered in very diluted forms and taken orally or sublingually.
- **How Nosodes Are Used**: Homeopaths may recommend nosodes as a preventive measure, similar to the concept

of "homeoprophylaxis," which involves giving a series of nosodes over time to boost immunity.

- **Effectiveness and Safety**: Nosodes have not undergone the same level of research as vaccines, and regulatory bodies like the FDA do not approve them as vaccine substitutes. They are primarily used as an adjunct to bolster immune response but should not be relied upon as the sole form of immunity without guidance from a healthcare provider.

3. Herbal and Nutritional Supplements for Immune Support

Herbal and nutritional supplements can be part of a holistic approach to supporting children's health. Certain herbs are known for their immune-supportive properties and may offer gentle protection during high-risk times.

- **Elderberry**: Known for its high antioxidant content, elderberry is commonly used during cold and flu seasons to boost immunity.
- **Echinacea**: This herb is often used at the onset of cold symptoms and is believed to enhance the immune system's ability to fight infection.
- **Vitamin D**: Essential for immune health, vitamin D is particularly beneficial during winter months when sun exposure is limited.
- **Vitamin C**: High doses of vitamin C are linked to immune health and may reduce the duration of colds and support faster recovery.

4. Homeoprophylaxis Protocols

Homeoprophylaxis (HP) is a homeopathic method of disease prevention, using highly diluted substances that mimic the disease they aim to prevent. Practitioners of HP suggest it can help build immunity without exposing the body to active pathogens.

- **How it Works**: HP uses a series of nosodes tailored to specific diseases and is often spread out over weeks or months. Practitioners believe this exposure helps the body recognize and respond to various pathogens, although HP is not universally accepted as a replacement for vaccines.
- **What to Expect**: HP protocols are usually overseen by a certified homeopath, and parents are given instructions for administering the nosodes at home.
- **Limitations and Cautions**: While some families find HP beneficial, the medical consensus does not recognize it as a replacement for vaccination. Always consult a trusted healthcare provider when considering HP.

5. Additional Preventive Health Practices

Holistic approaches to health can support a child's overall immune resilience, aiming to protect against infection without vaccination. These practices are valuable additions, whether or not families choose traditional immunization.

- **Daily Hygiene Habits**: Encouraging regular hand-washing, particularly before meals and after outdoor play, reduces the transmission of germs.
- **Reducing Environmental Toxins**: Avoiding chemical-heavy household cleaners, using air purifiers, and limiting exposure to pollutants helps maintain overall health, reducing the load on the immune system.
- **Stress Reduction**: Chronic stress can weaken the immune

system. Practices like breathing exercises, mindfulness, and outdoor play help reduce stress and promote immune health.

Important Note on Alternative Immunity Practices

While alternatives like nosodes and homeoprophylaxis may offer immune support, it's essential to consult with healthcare professionals to ensure safe practices. Traditional vaccines are designed to confer immunity in a manner that has been extensively researched and regulated. Families seeking alternatives are encouraged to do thorough research and work with qualified holistic practitioners to create the best plan for their children.

Supporting Children with ADHD, Autism, and Seizures: The Role of Diet, Vaccines, and Holistic Approaches

Conditions like ADHD, autism, and seizure disorders affect many children and bring unique health needs. While symptoms and challenges vary, diet and lifestyle adjustments can play a meaningful role in managing and supporting these conditions. For parents considering vaccinations and dietary choices, taking a comprehensive approach to holistic support can create a foundation for a child's health and wellness.

1. **ADHD (Attention-Deficit/Hyperactivity Disorder)**

- **Dietary Connections**: Diet can have a noticeable impact on ADHD symptoms. Reducing sugar intake, avoiding artificial additives, and incorporating omega-3 fatty acids (found in fish and seeds) may help with attention and mood. Some studies suggest eliminating potential allergens like gluten and dairy could be beneficial, as sensitivities can sometimes exacerbate hyperactivity.

- **Vaccine Considerations**: While no vaccines are proven to cause ADHD, some parents choose a modified or delayed schedule out of caution, particularly if a family history suggests susceptibility to behavioral or neurological conditions. Consultation with healthcare providers helps navigate choices based on individual needs.
- **Holistic Support**: In addition to dietary changes, regular physical activity and mindfulness exercises, such as deep breathing or meditation, can support children with ADHD by promoting self-regulation and reducing stress.

2. Autism Spectrum Disorder (ASD)

- **Diet and Gut Health**: Many parents of children with autism notice improvements in mood and behavior when addressing gut health. Probiotics, omega-3 fatty acids, and nutrient-dense foods like leafy greens and nuts support digestive health and may influence brain function. Diets free from gluten and casein (a protein found in dairy) are also sometimes used.
- **Vaccine Considerations**: While extensive studies have found no direct link between vaccines and autism, some parents consider adjusted vaccine schedules, especially if autism spectrum disorder runs in the family. Discussing options with a pediatrician familiar with ASD helps align vaccination choices with the child's health profile.
- **Holistic Support**: Sensory-friendly therapies, biofeedback, and energy-based practices like Reiki can help manage stress and improve mood, providing additional support to

children with autism.

3. Seizure Disorders

- **Ketogenic Diet and Nutritional Support**: The ketogenic diet (high fat, low carb) is sometimes used to help control seizures, as ketones produced by this diet may provide an alternative energy source for the brain. Supplements like magnesium and B vitamins are also supportive and may play a role in reducing seizure frequency.
- **Vaccine Considerations**: Some parents of children with seizure disorders prefer a modified vaccine approach, especially if certain vaccines have previously triggered seizures or febrile reactions. Collaborating with neurologists and pediatricians can help guide safe and personalized vaccination schedules.
- **Holistic Support**: Emerging research suggests CBD oil may support seizure management for some children, especially in cases resistant to traditional treatments. Other holistic practices, such as regular exercise and stress reduction techniques, are also beneficial.

Integrating Diet and Vaccine Decisions with Holistic Support

Taking a holistic approach to these conditions emphasizes individualized care and preventive health measures. Dietary choices and thoughtful vaccine considerations, combined with other supportive therapies, can empower parents to provide a comprehensive support system for their children.

Protecting Your Freedom of Choice

As a parent, you have the right to make informed decisions about your child's health, including whether or not to vaccinate. By understanding the exemption laws in your state, filing the necessary paperwork, and staying confident in your choices, you can navigate the school and daycare systems while honoring your family's health beliefs.

Informed decisions about vaccinations are critical. Every family's situation is unique, and it's essential to consider both personal experiences and the broader health implications when making decisions about vaccines. Whether you follow the standard schedule, delay certain vaccines, or explore alternative options, the most important thing is that you're making a choice based on what's best for your child.

This chapter reinforces the importance of exploring all health options within the crunchy lifestyle. Just as with food, natural remedies, and environmental choices, vaccinations are another area where parents can seek out information, ask questions, and make informed decisions that align with their family's values and health priorities.

In the next chapter, we'll dive into another critical aspect of holistic health: the hidden dangers of household toxins. We'll explore how to detoxify your home and life, making choices that protect your family's long-term wellness.

5

Detoxifying Your Life: Safe Products for Home and Body

Imagine your home as a sanctuary of well-being—a place where your family can thrive, free from harmful chemicals and toxins that disrupt health and harmony. We often think of our homes as safe spaces, but the truth is, many everyday products can introduce toxins into the air, water, and surfaces we touch. From cleaning supplies to personal care items, the ingredients in these products can have a long-term impact on our health, especially for young, developing children. Detoxifying your home and life is essential for creating a nurturing, balanced environment where your children can grow and thrive.

The importance of using non-toxic products to protect and promote family health cannot be overstated. As part of a holistic approach to parenting, detoxifying your life and home is a vital step in raising well-balanced children. This chapter explores how to identify common toxins and offers practical alternatives that will help you create a healthier, toxin-free environment for your family.

Identifying Common Toxins

We live in a world where convenience often comes at the cost of health. Many common household products contain chemicals that, over time, can have harmful effects on our bodies, especially for children who are still developing. Learning how to identify these toxins is the first step in making safer choices for your family.

Household Products to Watch Out For

Many household cleaning supplies, personal care products, and even furniture contain harmful chemicals that can disrupt health in subtle but cumulative ways. Here are some of the most common offenders:

- **Phthalates:** Found in many fragranced products, including air fresheners, soaps, and shampoos, phthalates are hormone disruptors that have been linked to reproductive issues and developmental problems in children.
- **Triclosan:** Often added to antibacterial soaps and hand sanitizers, triclosan has been shown to affect thyroid function and contribute to antibiotic resistance.
- **Formaldehyde:** Used in furniture, pressed wood products, and some nail polishes, formaldehyde is a known carcinogen that can cause respiratory irritation and allergic reactions.
- **Volatile Organic Compounds (VOCs):** Found in paint, carpet, and cleaning products, VOCs can cause headaches, respiratory issues, and long-term health effects, especially for those with asthma or allergies.
- **Parabens:** These preservatives, commonly found in personal care products like lotions and shampoos, are linked to hormonal imbalances and have been detected in breast cancer tissues.

Long-Term Health Impacts

The effects of cumulative exposure to these toxic chemicals can be particularly damaging for children, whose bodies are still growing and developing. Studies have shown that long-term exposure to toxins in household products can lead to respiratory issues, developmental delays, hormonal imbalances, and even chronic illnesses like asthma and allergies. Children are especially vulnerable because they tend to spend more time on the floor, put objects in their mouths, and are generally more sensitive to environmental toxins.

Over time, the build-up of chemicals in the body—known as body burden—can interfere with normal bodily functions and contribute to disease later in life. By reducing your family's exposure to harmful chemicals now, you can safeguard their long-term health and well-being.

Safer Alternatives

Once you become aware of the potential dangers lurking in your household products, the next step is to take action by switching to safer alternatives. Detoxifying your home doesn't need to happen overnight, but even small changes can make a big difference.

Non-Toxic Cleaning and Personal Care

Switching to non-toxic cleaning supplies and personal care products is one of the easiest and most impactful ways to reduce your family's exposure to harmful chemicals. Here are some simple swaps:

- **Vinegar and Baking Soda for Cleaning:** These two pantry staples can clean almost anything in your home, from counter tops to toilets, without introducing harmful chemicals into your environment.

- **Castile Soap:** A vegetable-based soap, castile is a great non-toxic option for hand washing, dish washing, and even cleaning floors.
- **Essential Oils:** Instead of using synthetic fragrances or air fresheners, essential oils like lavender, tea tree, and lemon can provide natural scents while offering antimicrobial properties.
- **Natural Lotions and Shampoos:** Look for products free from parabens, phthalates, and synthetic fragrances. Brands that focus on clean beauty and skincare offer safer alternatives that don't compromise on quality.

Creating a Safe Home Environment

Detoxifying your life goes beyond just cleaning products. Here are some practical tips for creating a healthier living space from top to bottom:

- **Air Purification:** Indoor air can often be more polluted than outdoor air, especially in homes with poor ventilation. Consider investing in air purifiers with HEPA filters, which can capture harmful particles like dust, mold, and VOCs. Opening windows regularly to allow fresh air to circulate is another simple yet effective way to improve indoor air quality.
- **Non-Toxic Furniture:** When possible, choose furniture made from solid wood rather than pressed wood, which often contains formaldehyde. Look for mattresses and couches made from organic materials that are free from flame retardants and other toxic chemicals.
- **Reducing Plastic Use:** Plastic containers can leach harmful chemicals, especially when heated. Replace plastic food

storage with glass or stainless steel alternatives. Reducing plastic use overall helps minimize your family's exposure to BPA and other plastic-related toxins.

Alternatives to Plastic Products

Reducing plastic use is not only beneficial for the environment but also for your family's health. Plastics can leach chemicals like BPA, phthalates, and other endocrine disruptors that may impact developing bodies. Here are some easy swaps to help create a safer, plastic-free environment for your family.

1. Food Storage Containers

- **Alternative**: Glass or Stainless Steel Containers
- **Why**: Glass and stainless steel are durable, don't retain odors, and are free from harmful chemicals that can leach into food.
- **Tip**: Look for glass containers with bamboo or silicone lids, which are more sustainable and still provide a good seal.

2. Water Bottles

- **Alternative**: Stainless Steel or Glass Bottles
- **Why**: These options don't leach chemicals, and stainless steel bottles are highly durable for on-the-go use.
- **Tip**: Choose insulated stainless steel bottles to keep water cool and reduce the need for disposable plastic bottles.

3. Food Wraps

- **Alternative**: Beeswax Wraps or Silicone Food Covers

- **Why**: Beeswax wraps are reusable, moldable, and can keep food fresh just like plastic wrap. Silicone covers are stretchable and easy to clean.
- **Tip**: Use beeswax wraps to cover bowls, wrap sandwiches, or store produce.

4. Kids' Tableware

- **Alternative**: Bamboo, Stainless Steel, or Silicone Plates and Utensils
- **Why**: These materials are durable, non-toxic, and better for the environment than disposable plastic options.
- **Tip**: Opt for bamboo plates and utensils for a lightweight, natural choice, or silicone if you want something soft and flexible for younger children.

5. Straws

- **Alternative**: Stainless Steel, Silicone, or Glass Straws
- **Why**: Reusable straws eliminate the need for single-use plastics and are safer for the environment.
- **Tip**: Stainless steel straws are durable and dishwasher-safe, while silicone straws are softer and better suited for younger children.

6. Cleaning Tools

- **Alternative**: Wooden Brushes with Natural Bristles or Metal Scrubbers
- **Why**: Wooden brushes and metal scrubbers are biodegradable or recyclable, and they last longer than plastic sponges.

- **Tip**: Look for dish brushes with replaceable heads, so you only need to replace the bristles rather than the whole brush.

7. Shopping Bags

- **Alternative**: Cloth Tote Bags and Mesh Produce Bags
- **Why**: Reusable bags reduce plastic waste, and mesh bags are ideal for fruits and vegetables.
- **Tip**: Keep a few reusable bags in your car or by the door so you always have them on hand for shopping trips.

8. Toothbrushes

- **Alternative**: Bamboo Toothbrushes
- **Why**: Bamboo is biodegradable, unlike plastic, and many bamboo toothbrushes now have recyclable bristles.
- **Tip**: Replace bamboo toothbrushes every 3-4 months, and compost the handle when done.

9. Baby Bottles

- **Alternative**: Glass or Stainless Steel Bottles
- **Why**: Glass and stainless steel are non-toxic and don't leach chemicals when warmed, unlike plastic bottles.
- **Tip**: Use silicone sleeves on glass bottles to prevent breakage, making them safer and more durable for little hands.

10. Toys

- **Alternative**: Wooden or Silicone Toys
- **Why**: Wooden toys are durable and made from natural

materials, while silicone toys are safe, soft, and free from harmful chemicals.

- **Tip**: Look for toys made with non-toxic paints and finishes, ensuring they're safe if your child puts them in their mouth.

Making the Transition to a Plastic-Free Home

Switching from plastic to alternative materials doesn't have to happen all at once. Start by swapping out items used frequently, like water bottles and food storage, and gradually work toward other changes. Every step you take to reduce plastic use creates a healthier home for your family and benefits the environment.

A Family's Journey to a Toxin-Free Home

The Parker family began their journey toward a toxin-free home after their youngest daughter was diagnosed with asthma. After months of relying on inhalers and medications, they started to wonder if something in their home environment was making her condition worse. They decided to eliminate synthetic cleaning products, swap out their plastic food containers, and invest in an air purifier. Within a few months, they noticed a significant improvement in their daughter's symptoms. She had fewer asthma attacks, slept better, and had more energy. The family now follows a non-toxic lifestyle and continues to make small changes to improve their home's environment.

A Case Study: Community Initiative for Toxin-Free Schools

In a small town in Vermont, a group of parents became concerned about the cleaning products being used in their children's school. After learning about the harmful effects of chemicals like ammonia and bleach, they rallied together to launch a "green cleaning" initiative. The parents worked with school administrators to replace toxic cleaning supplies with non-toxic, Eco-friendly alternatives. Within a year, the initiative expanded to include all schools in the district, improving the air quality and reducing exposure to chemicals for hundreds of children. The community's efforts not only benefited the students' health but also raised awareness about the importance of detoxifying public spaces.

Switching to non-toxic products not only safeguards your family's health but also supports a balanced, holistic lifestyle. Detoxifying your life allows you to create a healthier environment that promotes long-term well-being for your children. By making conscious choices, you're investing in your family's future health and nurturing a home that aligns with the principles of natural living.

By detoxifying your life, you align with the broader principles of holistic health. Every product you swap out for a safer alternative is a step toward creating an environment that fosters your children's natural growth and development. It's about making conscious choices that reflect your commitment to long-term wellness.

The next chapter delves into the fascinating world of gut health. We'll explore how the gut plays a central role in your child's overall wellness, impacting everything from immunity to emotional balance. Understanding and supporting gut health is key to raising healthy, well-balanced children.

Using Ozone Safely at Home

Ozone therapy has gained popularity for its potential benefits in air purification, water treatment, and therapeutic uses. Ozone (O_3) is a powerful oxidizer, often used to eliminate bacteria, viruses, mold, and other harmful particles. When used correctly, ozone can enhance home environments and promote health, but it's essential to follow safety guidelines, as exposure to high levels of ozone can be harmful.

Benefits of Ozone Use at Home

1. **Air Purification**: Ozone air purifiers break down airborne contaminants, neutralizing odors and killing bacteria and mold spores. This can improve air quality, especially in areas prone to high humidity or in homes with pets.
2. **Water Purification**: Ozone systems can be used to purify drinking water, disinfect surfaces, or treat bathwater. Ozone breaks down harmful microorganisms without leaving chemical residues, making it a natural alternative to traditional chemical disinfectants.
3. **Surface Sanitization**: Portable ozone generators can sanitize toys, furniture, and other surfaces. This is particularly beneficial for reducing allergens and germs in households with young children or individuals with respiratory sensitivities.

Safe Practices for Home Ozone Use

- **Proper Ventilation**: Always use ozone generators in well-ventilated areas. After running an ozone generator, wait before re-entering the space to allow ozone to break down into oxygen.
- **Time-Controlled Use**: Limit the duration of ozone exposure to prevent build-up. Most household ozone units have a timer function; follow the manufacturer's guidelines for safe operation.
- **Keep Away from People and Pets**: Ozone should not be

inhaled directly. When purifying air or surfaces, ensure people and pets are not in the room during treatment, and ventilate thoroughly afterward.

Household Applications of Ozone

- **Cleaning and Disinfecting Fruits and Vegetables**: Ozonated water can be used to clean produce, removing pesticides, bacteria, and other contaminants.
- **Laundry and Bathroom Use**: Ozonated water can replace some chemical disinfectants for washing clothes or sanitizing bathrooms.
- **Mold and Odor Removal**: Run ozone generators in closed-off spaces to treat mold, musty odors, and pet smells. For persistent mold issues, repeated treatments may be necessary.

Creating a Healthier Home with Steam, Humidifiers, Dehumidifiers, and Diffusers

Maintaining clean air and balanced humidity levels is essential for a healthy home, especially in spaces where children and family members with sensitivities spend a lot of time. Steam cleaners, humidifiers, dehumidifiers, and diffusers each play unique roles in reducing allergens, controlling moisture, and enhancing indoor air quality.

1. **Steam Cleaning for Chemical-Free Sanitization**

- **Benefits**: Steam cleaners use high-temperature steam to disinfect surfaces, eliminating bacteria, viruses, and dust mites without the need for chemical cleaners. This makes steam cleaning an excellent choice for homes with young children, pets, or those sensitive to cleaning chemicals.

- **Uses**: Steam cleaners are versatile, working well on floors, carpets, curtains, upholstery, grout, and bathroom surfaces. They also help eliminate dust mites, a common allergen.
- **Safe Practices**: After steam cleaning, allow surfaces to dry completely, particularly on fabrics or porous materials, to prevent mold and mildew growth.

2. Humidifiers for Dry Indoor Air

- **Benefits**: Humidifiers add moisture to dry air, which can help alleviate respiratory issues, reduce skin dryness, and prevent the spread of certain airborne viruses. They are especially beneficial in winter when heating systems dry out indoor air.
- **Types**: Choose from cool-mist, warm-mist, or ultrasonic humidifiers. Cool-mist models are safe for kids' rooms, while warm-mist models can help with congestion.
- **Safe Practices**: Regularly clean humidifiers to prevent mold and bacterial growth. Use distilled water to minimize mineral deposits and aim for a humidity level between 30-50% to avoid excess moisture.

3. Dehumidifiers for Damp Environments

- **Benefits**: Dehumidifiers reduce excess moisture, which is essential in humid climates or areas prone to dampness, like basements. Lowering humidity levels helps prevent mold and dust mites, improving air quality and reducing musty odors.

- **Uses**: Ideal for areas with high humidity, dehumidifiers can help prevent mold-related health issues and improve comfort, especially during summer months.
- **Safe Practices**: Empty and clean the water reservoir regularly to prevent bacterial growth. Aim for an indoor humidity level of 30-50%, adjusting seasonally to maintain comfort and reduce mold risk.

4. Essential Oil Diffusers for Air Quality and Wellness

- **Benefits**: Diffusers disperse essential oils into the air, adding a pleasant aroma while also offering therapeutic benefits. Many essential oils, such as lavender and eucalyptus, are known for their calming and purifying properties, which can help reduce stress, promote sleep, or aid in respiratory health.
- **Types**: Ultrasonic diffusers are popular, creating a fine mist without heating the oils, which helps preserve their therapeutic qualities. Nebulizing diffusers, which use air to break down the oil, are ideal for stronger scent diffusion without added moisture.
- **Safe Practices**: When using around children, ensure oils are safe and kid-friendly (e.g., lavender, chamomile). Avoid potent oils like peppermint or eucalyptus with young children, and never leave a diffuser running unattended. Limit diffusion to 15-30 minutes in a closed room to avoid overwhelming scents.

5. Balancing Humidity and Air Quality

- **Why It Matters**: Proper humidity (30-50%) promotes

respiratory health, reduces skin irritation, and minimizes static electricity. It also prevents conditions favorable to mold growth. Regularly monitoring humidity with a hygrometer can help you determine when to use a humidifier or dehumidifier.

- **Daily Practice**: Use these tools as needed based on seasonal conditions, humidity levels, and your family's health needs, creating an optimal indoor environment year-round.

Using Essential Oils at Home: Diffusion, Safety, and Natural Cleaning

Essential oils offer a versatile and natural way to create a healthier home environment. From adding pleasant aromas to your home to serving as natural cleaning agents, essential oils have many uses. Here's a quick guide on safely diffusing oils, choosing safe oils for your family, and using them as Eco-friendly cleaners.

1. **Diffusing Essential Oils for Wellness and Calm**

- **Benefits**: Diffusing essential oils can enhance mood, reduce stress, improve focus, and support respiratory health. Popular options like lavender, chamomile, and eucalyptus have calming or purifying effects.
- **How to Diffuse**: Use an ultrasonic or nebulizing diffuser, following the manufacturer's instructions. For a gentle diffusion, add 5-10 drops to the diffuser's water reservoir.
- **Recommended Usage**: Limit diffusion to 15-30 minutes in a closed room to avoid overpowering the scent, especially around young children or pets.

2. Essential Oil Safety Tips

- **Dilution**: Essential oils are highly concentrated, so always dilute with a carrier oil (like coconut or almond oil) if applying to skin. Use 1-2 drops per tablespoon of carrier oil for children.
- **Kid-Friendly Oils**: Safe options for kids include lavender, chamomile, and orange. Avoid peppermint, eucalyptus, and tea tree oils around infants and young children, as these can be too potent for their sensitive systems.
- **Avoid Ingestion**: Essential oils should generally not be ingested, as they are not regulated for internal use and can be toxic in concentrated forms. Stick to external use or diffusion for safe home use.

3. Using Essential Oils as Natural Cleaners

- **Benefits**: Essential oils like lemon, tea tree, and lavender have natural antibacterial, antiviral, and anti fungal properties, making them effective in cleaning.
- **DIY Cleaner Recipes**:
- **All-Purpose Cleaner**: Mix 1 cup of white vinegar, 1 cup of water, and 10-15 drops of lemon or tea tree oil. This works well on counter tops, sinks, and glass surfaces.
- **Disinfecting Spray**: Combine 1 cup of water, 1 cup of rubbing alcohol, and 10 drops of lavender or eucalyptus oil for a natural disinfectant.
- **Usage**: Store your cleaners in spray bottles, and shake before each use to disperse the oils evenly. Essential oils add a pleasant scent and boost cleaning power without harsh chemicals.

10 Natural Cleaner Recipes

Switching to natural, non-toxic cleaners is one of the easiest ways to detoxify your home and create a safer environment for your family. Here are 10 simple DIY recipes to replace common household cleaners with Eco-friendly, effective alternatives.

1. All-Purpose Cleaner

This cleaner works on most surfaces, from counter tops to bathroom tiles.

Ingredients:

- 1 cup distilled water
- 1 cup white vinegar
- 10 drops of lemon essential oil (for scent and added cleaning power)
- 10 drops of tea tree essential oil (for antibacterial properties)

Instructions:

1. Combine all ingredients in a spray bottle.
2. Shake well before use. Spray on surfaces and wipe with a clean cloth.

2. Glass and Mirror Cleaner

Get streak-free mirrors and windows without the harsh chemicals.

Ingredients:

- 1 cup distilled water
- 1 cup white vinegar

- 2 tablespoons rubbing alcohol
- 5 drops of peppermint or lemon essential oil (optional, for scent)

Instructions:

1. Mix ingredients in a spray bottle.
2. Spray directly onto glass surfaces and wipe with a microfiber cloth for a streak-free shine.
3. **Natural Floor Cleaner**

This is safe for hardwood, laminate, and tile floors.

Ingredients:

- 1 gallon warm water
- ½ cup white vinegar
- 5-10 drops of your favorite essential oil (e.g., lavender, eucalyptus, or orange)

Instructions:

1. Mix vinegar and essential oil in the warm water.
2. Mop as usual. Allow floors to air dry—no need to rinse.

4. Disinfecting Bathroom Cleaner

A powerful cleaner for the bathroom that tackles germs and grime.

Ingredients:

- ½ cup baking soda
- ¼ cup liquid castile soap

- 1 tablespoon hydrogen peroxide
- 10 drops tea tree oil (for disinfecting)
- 10 drops eucalyptus oil (for fresh scent)

Instructions:

1. Mix the ingredients into a thick paste.
2. Apply to bathroom surfaces like sinks, tubs, and toilets using a sponge. Let it sit for a few minutes, then scrub and rinse.

5. Natural Toilet Bowl Cleaner

A simple yet effective toilet cleaner with natural ingredients.

Ingredients:

- ½ cup baking soda
- ½ cup white vinegar
- 10 drops tea tree essential oil (optional)

Instructions:

1. Sprinkle the baking soda into the toilet bowl.
2. Pour in the vinegar and let it fizz for a few minutes.
3. Scrub with a toilet brush, then flush.

6. Carpet Freshener

Deodorize carpets and rugs with this simple recipe.

Ingredients:

- 1 cup baking soda
- 10-15 drops of lavender or eucalyptus essential oil

Instructions:

1. Combine baking soda and essential oil in a jar. Shake well.
2. Sprinkle lightly over carpets. Let it sit for 15-20 minutes, then vacuum.

7. Furniture Polish

Keep wood furniture looking fresh and polished.

Ingredients:

- 1/4 cup olive oil
- 1/4 cup white vinegar
- 10 drops lemon essential oil

Instructions:

1. Mix ingredients in a small bowl or jar.
2. Use a soft cloth to apply the polish to wood furniture. Buff with a dry cloth until it shines.

8. Stainless Steel Cleaner

A natural cleaner to keep stainless steel appliances fingerprint-free.

Ingredients:

- 1/2 cup white vinegar
- 1/2 cup water
- 1 tablespoon olive oil

Instructions:

1. Combine vinegar and water in a spray bottle.
2. Spray on stainless steel surfaces and wipe with a microfiber cloth.
3. Add a few drops of olive oil to the cloth to buff the surface and prevent future fingerprints.

9. Natural Air Freshener Spray

Freshen your home with a simple, chemical-free air freshener.

Ingredients:

- 1 cup distilled water
- 1 tablespoon baking soda
- 10-15 drops of your favorite essential oil (lavender, lemon, or orange)

Instructions:

1. Mix all ingredients in a spray bottle.
2. Shake well before use and spritz around your home as needed.

10. Dishwasher Detergent

A simple powder that works in place of commercial dishwasher detergents.

Ingredients:

- 1 cup washing soda
- 1 cup baking soda
- ½ cup citric acid
- ½ cup coarse sea salt

Instructions:

1. Combine all ingredients in an airtight container.
2. Use 1–2 tablespoons of the powder per dishwasher load. For added shine, you can also add white vinegar to the rinse aid compartment.

Natural Cleaning for a Healthier Home

By using these natural, DIY cleaning alternatives, you can drastically reduce your family's exposure to toxic chemicals while still maintaining a clean and fresh home. Each recipe is simple, cost-effective, and aligned with a holistic, Eco-friendly lifestyle.

6

Hidden Health Threats: Parasites, Mold, Heavy Metals, Candida, and Lyme Disease

In the quest for better health, we often focus on nutrition, exercise, and lifestyle changes, but there are deeper, hidden health threats that can disrupt wellness in profound ways. Parasites, mold, heavy metals, candida overgrowth, and Lyme disease can silently impact your health and your child's development, leading to chronic symptoms that are often misdiagnosed or overlooked. By understanding and addressing these issues holistically, you can take control of your family's health, tackling the root causes of various ailments.

Understanding Root Causes: The Basis of Illness and Imbalance

When it comes to health, addressing symptoms alone often leads to temporary relief but doesn't tackle the underlying issues that cause chronic problems. The concept of root causes is fundamental in holistic health and emphasizes identifying and treating the deeper reasons behind ailments rather than just their symptoms.

What Are Root Causes?

Root causes refer to the underlying factors that contribute to illness or imbalance in the body. These can include dietary deficiencies, chronic stress, environmental toxins, gut health issues, poor lifestyle habits, and even emotional trauma. By focusing on these elements, it's possible to build a comprehensive approach to restoring and maintaining health.

Why Root Causes Matter

Addressing root causes is essential for long-term health and well-being. When the true source of an issue is identified, treatment becomes more effective, and healing can be more lasting. Oftentimes, allopathic medicine treats the symptoms covering up the underlying root cause. For instance, recurring digestive issues may not just be due to poor diet but could stem from imbalances in gut bacteria, stress, or hidden food intolerances. Similarly, skin problems like eczema might be linked to gut health, liver function, or exposure to toxins.

Common Root Causes and Their Impact

1. **Gut Health Imbalances**: The gut is often called the "second brain" because of its critical role in overall health. Imbalances in gut bacteria can lead to inflammation, weakened

immunity, and even mood disorders due to disrupted neurotransmitter production.

2. **Nutrient Deficiencies**: Insufficient levels of vitamins and minerals can lead to a range of health issues, from poor energy levels and weakened immune response to developmental delays in children.
3. **Toxin Exposure**: Continuous exposure to environmental toxins—like chemicals in household products, pesticides, or heavy metals—can overwhelm the body's detoxification system, leading to chronic fatigue, hormonal imbalances, or cognitive issues.
4. **Chronic Stress**: Persistent stress can negatively impact the body by disrupting hormone balance, depleting vital nutrients, and impairing digestion, making it a significant root cause of health problems.
5. **Emotional and Psychological Factors**: Emotional trauma and unresolved stress can manifest physically, leading to conditions such as headaches, digestive disturbances, and autoimmune issues.
6. **Lifestyle Factors**: Poor sleep, a sedentary lifestyle, and insufficient hydration contribute to systemic inflammation and reduced body function.

A Holistic Approach to Addressing Root Causes

In holistic health, identifying and addressing these root causes involves looking at the whole picture—diet, lifestyle, environment, and emotional health. For example:

- **Improving Gut Health**: Incorporating probiotics, fermented foods, and a diet rich in fiber can help restore gut flora balance.

- **Reducing Toxin Exposure**: Switching to non-toxic household products and paying attention to clean, organic food choices can help reduce the toxic burden on the body.
- **Managing Stress**: Techniques like mindfulness, yoga, and deep breathing exercises aid in regulating stress and promoting a balanced nervous system.
- **Supplementing Wisely**: Using targeted supplements, such as magnesium, omega-3s, and vitamin D, can address deficiencies and support overall wellness.

The Power of Prevention

Understanding root causes also opens the door to prevention. When parents incorporate practices that address potential root causes—like a nutrient-dense diet, reducing toxin exposure, and promoting emotional well-being—they help create a solid foundation for their children's long-term health.

Parasites: The Silent Saboteurs

Parasites are more prevalent than many people realize, particularly in children who are frequently exposed to outdoor environments, pets, and public spaces. These microscopic or larger organisms live inside the body, feeding off essential nutrients and often causing a range of subtle to severe symptoms. The impact of parasites can extend beyond digestive discomfort to affect immunity, energy levels, and even behavior.

Signs of Parasite Infection

- **Unexplained Digestive Issues**: Symptoms such as bloating, gas, constipation, or diarrhea that persist without a clear cause.

- **Chronic Fatigue or Irritability**: A constant sense of tiredness that does not improve with rest, often paired with mood swings or increased irritability.
- **Itchy Skin or Rashes**: Unexplained itching, hives, or rashes that come and go without an obvious trigger.
- **Bruxism (Teeth Grinding)**: Grinding teeth during sleep, which may be a response to discomfort caused by parasites.
- **Changes in Appetite**: Sudden increases or decreases in appetite, often accompanied by strong cravings for sweets or processed carbohydrates.
- **Nutritional Deficiencies**: Despite a balanced diet, persistent nutrient deficiencies can be an indicator that parasites are absorbing the nutrients the body needs.

Holistic Approach to Managing Parasites

Herbal Remedies:

- **Wormwood**: Known for its powerful anti parasitic properties, wormwood contains compounds that can help weaken and expel parasites from the body.
- **Black Walnut**: Traditionally used to treat parasitic infections, black walnut hulls are rich in juglone, which creates an environment that is hostile to parasites.
- **Clove**: This herb not only helps kill adult parasites but also destroys parasite eggs, preventing the cycle from continuing. Including clove as part of a comprehensive detox protocol is essential for effective parasite cleansing.
- **Oregano Oil**: A natural antimicrobial that can be effective against various parasites and pathogens when used properly.

Dietary Support:

- **Reduce Sugar and Processed Foods**: Parasites thrive on sugar and refined carbohydrates. Reducing these foods helps starve them and supports a healthier gut environment.
- **Increase Fiber Intake**: Foods high in fiber help flush out parasites by supporting regular bowel movements and maintaining gut health.
- **Garlic**: This powerful natural anti parasitic has sulfur-containing compounds that can aid in expelling parasites. Adding raw or cooked garlic to meals can provide ongoing support.
- **Pumpkin Seeds**: Rich in compounds called cucurbitins, pumpkin seeds paralyze parasites, making it easier for the body to eliminate them.
- **Papaya Seeds**: Containing enzymes like papain, papaya seeds can help break down parasite protein structures and assist in their removal from the digestive system.

Probiotic Support:

- **Rebuilding Gut Flora**: After a parasite cleanse, introducing high-quality probiotics helps replenish beneficial gut bacteria, restoring balance and improving digestion and immunity.

Additional Remedies:

- **Activated Charcoal**: Can bind to toxins and parasite waste products, aiding in their removal from the body.
- **Apple Cider Vinegar**: The acidity of apple cider vinegar can

make the digestive system less hospitable to parasites.

- **Fennel**: This herb not only aids digestion but also has mild anti parasitic properties that can support gut health.

Prevention and Maintenance

- **Good Hygiene Practices**: Regular hand washing, especially after playing outside, using the bathroom, or handling pets, is essential.
- **Routine Deworming**: For families with pets or frequent outdoor exposure, regular deworming protocols can be beneficial.
- **Thoroughly Washing Produce**: Ensuring that fruits and vegetables are cleaned properly to remove any potential parasites or eggs.

By incorporating these holistic practices and remedies, parents can support their child's health and create an environment that helps prevent and manage parasitic infections naturally. Addressing parasite health not only improves physical well-being but can also have a positive impact on mood, energy levels, and cognitive function.

Mold: A Hidden Home Invader

Mold exposure is often overlooked but can have significant and lasting effects on respiratory, immune, and overall health. Mold thrives in damp, humid environments, and its spores can release harmful mycotoxins into the air. These toxins are known to contribute to respiratory issues, cognitive difficulties, and chronic fatigue, making it essential for parents to be aware of and address mold exposure, especially for the well-being of children.

Signs of Mold Exposure

- **Frequent Sinus Infections or Respiratory Problems**: Persistent nasal congestion, sneezing, and respiratory discomfort are common signs.
- **Chronic Cough or Wheezing**: A dry, unexplained cough or wheezing that worsens indoors may indicate mold exposure.
- **Fatigue, Brain Fog, or Headaches**: Mold toxins can impair cognitive function, leading to difficulties in concentration, memory issues, and chronic headaches.
- **Unexplained Skin Rashes**: Red, itchy, or inflamed skin that isn't attributed to allergies or known irritants.
- **Heightened Allergy Symptoms**: Increased sensitivity to allergens, particularly when indoors, may suggest mold presence.

Holistic Approach to Mold Management

Air Quality Control:

- **Air Purifiers**: Invest in high-quality HEPA air purifiers to help capture mold spores and improve indoor air quality.
- **Dehumidifiers**: Maintaining indoor humidity below 50% can inhibit mold growth. Dehumidifiers can be used in basements, bathrooms, and other moisture-prone areas to keep humidity levels in check.
- **Essential Oils**: Use tea tree oil or eucalyptus oil in diffusers, as they have natural anti fungal properties that can help reduce airborne mold spores.

Natural Cleaning Solutions:

- **Vinegar**: White vinegar can be an effective mold killer. Spray undiluted vinegar on moldy areas, let it sit for an hour, and wipe clean.
- **Tea Tree Oil**: A natural antiseptic, tea tree oil can be mixed with water (1 teaspoon per cup of water) and sprayed on affected areas to inhibit mold growth.

Detoxification Support:

- **Activated Charcoal**: Helps bind mycotoxins in the body, supporting their elimination and reducing toxin load.
- **Chlorella**: A natural algae that binds to heavy metals and toxins, aiding in the detoxification process.
- **Garlic**: Contains anti fungal properties and supports the immune system in combating mold exposure.
- **Probiotics**: Strengthen the gut microbiome, which plays a crucial role in overall immune response and helps the body combat mycotoxins more effectively.

Prevention Tips:

- **Repair Leaks Promptly**: Ensure that any leaks in the roof, plumbing, or windows are repaired quickly to prevent water damage and mold growth.
- **Good Ventilation**: Install exhaust fans in bathrooms and kitchens and open windows regularly to promote airflow and reduce moisture buildup.
- **Use Mold-Resistant Products**: Consider using mold-resistant drywall or paint in areas prone to moisture.

- **Monitor Humidity Levels**: Use a hygrometer to keep track of indoor humidity and ensure it remains below 50%.

By addressing mold proactively and supporting your body's detoxification, you can create a safer, healthier environment for your children. Managing mold exposure holistically not only improves respiratory health but also boosts energy levels and cognitive function, helping your family thrive.

Heavy Metal Toxicity: The Hidden Toxins in Our Environment

Heavy metals, including mercury, lead, arsenic, cadmium, and aluminum, are pervasive in our environment and can accumulate in the body over time. Exposure to these metals comes from various sources such as contaminated water, industrial pollution, certain foods, and household products. Chronic exposure to heavy metals can have a significant impact on health, affecting brain function, immune health, and energy levels. Children are particularly vulnerable to heavy metal toxicity, which can contribute to developmental delays, learning difficulties, and behavioral issues.

Types of Heavy Metals and Their Effects

1. **Mercury**:

- **Sources**: Found in some seafood (e.g., tuna, swordfish), dental amalgams, and industrial emissions.
- **Health Effects**: Mercury exposure can impair cognitive function, leading to memory issues, brain fog, and developmental delays in children. It can also affect motor skills and contribute to mood disorders.

2. **Lead**:

- **Sources**: Present in old paint, contaminated water supplies, certain toys, and soil.
- **Health Effects**: Lead toxicity can cause significant harm to the brain and nervous system, particularly in children. It is linked to cognitive deficits, attention disorders, and delayed growth and development.

3. **Arsenic**:

- **Sources**: Found in contaminated groundwater, rice products, and certain pesticides.
- **Health Effects**: Chronic arsenic exposure can lead to skin changes, digestive issues, and impaired cognitive function. High levels may also increase the risk of certain cancers.

4. **Cadmium**:

- **Sources**: Present in cigarette smoke, contaminated food (e.g., leafy greens, shellfish), and some industrial processes.
- **Health Effects**: Cadmium can accumulate in the kidneys and liver, leading to organ damage. It is also associated with bone demineralization and immune system suppression.

5. **Aluminum**:

- **Sources**: Common in cookware, certain vaccines, deodorants, and processed foods.
- **Health Effects**: Aluminum exposure has been linked to neurotoxicity and conditions like Alzheimer's disease. In

children, it can contribute to developmental delays and cognitive issues.

Signs of Heavy Metal Toxicity

- **Chronic Fatigue or Weakness**: Persistent tiredness that is not alleviated by rest.
- **Cognitive Problems**: Memory loss, brain fog, and difficulty concentrating.
- **Mood Swings or Irritability**: Unexplained mood changes or emotional instability.
- **Delayed Development or Behavioral Issues**: Learning difficulties, attention disorders, or developmental delays in children.

Holistic Approach to Managing Heavy Metal Toxicity
Chelation Therapy:

- **Natural Chelators**: Cilantro, chlorella, and zeolite are known for their ability to bind to heavy metals and facilitate their safe elimination from the body. Incorporating these natural chelators into a detox protocol can be effective for reducing heavy metal load.

Dietary Support:

- **Antioxidant-Rich Foods**: Foods high in antioxidants help neutralize the oxidative stress caused by heavy metals. Blueberries, spinach, turmeric, and green tea are excellent choices to support the detoxification process and protect cellular health.

- **Sulfur-Rich Foods**: Garlic, onions, and cruciferous vegetables (e.g., broccoli, cauliflower) help boost the body's detox pathways.

Supplemental Support:

- **Activated Charcoal**: Binds to toxins in the digestive system and aids in their removal.
- **Glutathione**: This powerful antioxidant helps neutralize free radicals and supports liver function, playing a crucial role in detoxification.
- **Probiotics**: Maintaining a healthy gut flora supports the body's natural ability to excrete toxins and enhances overall immune function.

Avoidance Strategies:

- **Reduce Exposure**: Opt for aluminum-free deodorants and cookware. Filter drinking water to remove heavy metals, and be mindful of food sources that may contain higher levels of contamination.
- **Limit Processed Foods**: Choose organic and whole foods when possible to minimize exposure to additives and contaminants.

Prevention and Ongoing Maintenance

- **Regular Testing**: Consider hair or urine analysis to monitor heavy metal levels, especially if exposure is suspected.
- **Safe Detox Practices**: Engage in periodic, gentle detox routines that include chelating herbs and supplements to

maintain low levels of heavy metals in the body.

- **Healthy Lifestyle Choices**: Encourage outdoor play and exercise to promote sweating, which is a natural way for the body to expel toxins.

By understanding the sources and effects of heavy metal exposure and incorporating holistic practices, parents can take proactive steps to protect their children's health. Supporting detoxification and minimizing exposure ensures that children can grow and thrive without the burden of hidden environmental toxins.

Candida Overgrowth: The Hidden Yeast

Candida is a type of yeast that naturally resides in the gut and contributes to healthy digestion and nutrient absorption. However, when it overgrows due to factors such as a poor diet, frequent use of antibiotics, high stress levels, or a weakened immune system, it can disrupt the natural balance and lead to various health issues. Candida overgrowth can manifest in a wide range of symptoms that impact both physical and mental well-being. Candida thrives on sugar and refined carbohydrates, making dietary choices a crucial aspect of controlling its proliferation.

Signs of Candida Overgrowth

- **Digestive Problems**: Bloating, gas, constipation, or diarrhea that persist without an obvious cause.
- **Strong Sugar Cravings**: A persistent desire for sweets and refined carbohydrates, which feed candida and fuel its growth.

- **Brain Fog or Memory Issues**: Difficulty focusing, poor memory, and overall cognitive sluggishness.
- **Recurring Yeast Infections or Skin Rashes**: Regular occurrences of thrush, athlete's foot, diaper rash, or fungal skin infections.
- **Mood Swings or Irritability**: Emotional instability, anxiety, and irritability that seem unrelated to external factors.
- **Chronic Fatigue**: Persistent low energy levels that do not improve with rest.

Holistic Approach to Managing Candida Overgrowth

1. **Dietary Changes**:

- **Reduce Sugar and Refined Carbohydrates**: Candida feeds on sugars and processed foods. Reducing or eliminating these from the diet is critical to starving the yeast and regaining balance.
- **Incorporate Anti-Candida Foods**: Focus on incorporating foods that help restore gut balance, such as leafy greens, non-starchy vegetables, lean proteins, and healthy fats like avocados and olive oil.
- **Increase Fiber Intake**: High-fiber foods help improve digestion and eliminate toxins, supporting the removal of excess candida from the body. Flax seeds, chia seeds, and leafy greens are great sources.

2. **Herbal and Natural Antifungals**:

- **Garlic**: Known for its powerful anti fungal and immune-boosting properties, garlic can be added to meals or taken as a supplement.

- **Coconut Oil**: Contains caprylic acid, which has natural anti fungal properties. Consuming a teaspoon daily or using it in cooking can help fight candida.
- **Oregano Oil**: A potent natural anti fungal, oregano oil can be taken in diluted form or in capsule form to target candida.
- **Pau d'Arco Tea**: This herbal tea has anti fungal properties that help combat candida overgrowth and support gut health.

3. **Probiotic and Gut Health Support**:

- **Probiotic-Rich Foods**: Consuming foods like sauerkraut, kimchi, kefir, and unsweetened yogurt introduces beneficial bacteria that help balance the gut microbiome.
- **Prebiotics**: Foods rich in prebiotics, such as garlic, onions, and bananas, help nourish the beneficial bacteria in the gut and support their growth.
- **Probiotic Supplements**: High-quality probiotics containing strains like *Lactobacillus* and *Bifidobacterium* can help restore the balance of good bacteria and curb candida overgrowth.

4. **Natural Detoxification Support**:

- **Activated Charcoal**: Helps bind toxins released by dying candida and aids in their removal from the body.
- **Chlorella**: A natural detoxifier that binds to heavy metals and toxins, supporting liver health and aiding in overall detoxification.
- **Lemon Water**: Drinking warm lemon water in the morning can help stimulate the liver and support detoxification processes.

5. Lifestyle Adjustments:

- **Manage Stress**: High stress levels can compromise the immune system and make it easier for candida to thrive. Incorporate mindfulness practices, deep breathing exercises, and regular physical activity to manage stress.
- **Prioritize Sleep**: Adequate sleep supports immune function and overall health, making it easier for the body to fight off candida overgrowth.

By implementing these holistic practices, parents can support their child's body in combating candida overgrowth, ensuring better digestion, improved energy levels, and enhanced overall well-being. Proper management of candida can lead to noticeable improvements in behavior, mood, and physical health.

Lyme Disease and Co-infections: A Complex Condition

Lyme disease, primarily transmitted through the bite of infected black-legged ticks (often called deer ticks), is becoming increasingly prevalent and poses significant challenges due to its multifaceted nature. The infection can lead to a wide range of symptoms, including chronic fatigue, joint pain, and cognitive impairments. A major complication with Lyme disease is that it frequently comes with co-infections, which can exacerbate symptoms and make diagnosis and treatment more complex.

How Lyme Disease is Transferred

Lyme disease is caused by the *Borrelia burgdorferi* bacterium, which is introduced into the bloodstream through tick bites. Ticks acquire the bacteria by feeding on infected animals such as deer and rodents. When they bite a human, they transmit the bacteria into the bloodstream, initiating the infection.

The Unreliable Deerborn Test for Lyme Disease

The conventional diagnostic test for Lyme disease, often referred to as the Deerborn test (Western blot and ELISA), has proven unreliable. This is primarily because individuals with chronic Lyme disease often do not produce sufficient antibodies for detection. The *OspA* vaccine further complicated testing reliability, as it targeted the outer surface protein A of the *Borrelia* bacterium, resulting in diagnostic inconsistencies. This has led to many cases of Lyme disease going undiagnosed or misdiagnosed, leaving individuals to suffer prolonged symptoms without effective treatment. The test has not been updated since its release in 1974 where they also declared that the individual must have an arthritic knee, because they knew at the time that the OspA vaccine worked best on individuals that had an arthritic knee. Please note the vaccine is no longer on the market as it was proven to spread Lyme Disease.

Signs of Lyme Disease

- **Chronic Fatigue and Weakness**: Persistent exhaustion that does not improve with rest.
- **Migratory Joint Pain**: Pain that shifts from one joint to another, often mistaken for other conditions.
- **Cognitive Issues**: Brain fog, memory problems, or difficulty focusing.
- **Unexplained Mood Swings or Anxiety**: Emotional instability that can appear unrelated to external factors.
- **Rashes or Skin Irritations**: The classic "bull's-eye" rash (erythema migrans) may or may not be present.

Co-infections Commonly Associated with Lyme Disease

Lyme disease rarely comes alone; it is often accompanied by co-infections that complicate the clinical picture. These include:

1. **Babesia**: A malaria-like parasite that infects red blood cells, leading to symptoms like fever, chills, and severe fatigue.
2. **Bartonella**: Known for causing symptoms such as swollen lymph nodes, neurological issues, and skin rashes.
3. **Ehrlichia/Anaplasma**: Bacteria that can lead to flu-like symptoms, including high fever and severe headaches.
4. **Mycoplasma**: A bacteria that can cause respiratory issues, joint pain, and chronic fatigue.
5. **Rickettsia**: Often associated with spotted fevers, it can lead to symptoms like rash, fever, and muscle pain.
6. **Tick-Borne Relapsing Fever (TBRF)**: Characterized by recurring episodes of fever, muscle aches, and fatigue.
7. **Chlamydia pneumoniae**: Linked to persistent respiratory symptoms and chronic fatigue.
8. **Toxoplasmosis**: A parasitic infection that can cause neurological symptoms and fatigue.
9. **Candida overgrowth**: Although not directly transmitted by ticks, candida often flourishes in individuals with weakened immune systems, compounding the severity of symptoms.

The Impact of Antibiotics on Co-infections

While antibiotics are the standard treatment for Lyme disease, they can sometimes worsen co-infections. Prolonged antibiotic use can disrupt the gut microbiome, leading to issues such as candida overgrowth and decreased immune function. This can make co-infections more persistent and harder to manage.

Holistic Approach to Managing Lyme Disease and Co-infections

Herbal Protocols:

- **Cat's Claw**: Known for its immune-boosting properties, cat's claw can help reduce inflammation and combat *Borrelia.*
- **Japanese Knotweed**: Contains resveratrol, which supports immune function and reduces inflammation.
- **Astragalus**: Helps fortify the immune system and is particularly effective during early stages of Lyme disease.
- **Cryptolepis and Sida acuta**: Effective against co-infections such as Babesia and Bartonella.

Biofeedback and Energy Medicine:

- **Biofeedback**: This technology can help detect the frequencies of Lyme and its co-infections, offering a non-invasive way to assess the body's condition.
- **Energy Medicine**: Techniques like Reiki and frequency therapy can help restore balance and promote healing within the body.

Detox Support:

- **Infrared Saunas**: Promote sweating, which aids in the removal of toxins released by Lyme bacteria and co-infections.
- **Lymphatic Drainage**: Gentle massage techniques to support lymph flow and reduce the toxin load in the body.
- **Detox Diets**: Incorporating foods rich in antioxidants, such as berries, leafy greens, and cruciferous vegetables, helps

the body combat oxidative stress.

- **Activated Charcoal and Bentonite Clay**: These binders help capture and eliminate toxins from the digestive tract.

By adopting a comprehensive approach that includes herbal support, energy medicine, and detox strategies, individuals can manage Lyme disease and its co-infections more effectively. This multifaceted approach helps reduce symptoms, boost immune health, and promote overall well-being.

Addressing Underlying Health Issues Holistically

These hidden health threats—parasites, mold, heavy metals, candida, and Lyme disease—can profoundly impact your family's health, often going unnoticed until symptoms become chronic. By taking a holistic approach and addressing these issues at their root, you can create a strong foundation of health for your children and yourself. Whether through diet, natural remedies, or detox protocols, tackling these underlying health problems can lead to a significant improvement in overall wellness.

7

The Gut Connection: Holistic Digestive Health

The gut, often referred to as the "second brain," plays a far more significant role in your child's overall health than most people realize. It's not just responsible for digesting food; the gut is central to regulating the immune system, balancing mood, and even supporting cognitive function. With trillions of bacteria living within the digestive tract, this "microbiome" communicates directly with the brain, influencing everything from behavior to emotional health. A healthy gut lays the foundation for raising well-balanced, thriving children.

Gut health is foundational to raising healthy, well-balanced children. It affects physical development, emotional regulation, mental clarity, and overall wellness. In this chapter, we'll explore the crucial role the gut plays in your child's life and how holistic strategies can support and enhance gut health for optimal well-being.

The Gut-Brain Axis

How Gut Health Impacts Behavior and Mood

The connection between the gut and the brain, known as

the gut-brain axis, is one of the most fascinating aspects of modern health research. The gut microbiome—composed of trillions of bacteria, fungi, and other microorganisms—has a direct line of communication with the brain, largely through the vagus nerve. This communication influences the production of neurotransmitters like serotonin, dopamine, and GABA, which play critical roles in regulating mood, behavior, and even sleep.

For children, gut health can have a profound impact on emotional regulation and cognitive function. Disruptions in the gut, such as an imbalance in the gut microbiota (dysbiosis), have been linked to a range of issues including anxiety, depression, hyperactivity, and even conditions like ADHD. When the gut is healthy and balanced, it supports the production of "feel-good" neurotransmitters, helping children feel more emotionally stable and focused.

Recognizing Gut Issues in Children

Digestive imbalances can manifest in various ways, and children often show gut health issues not just through physical symptoms but also behavioral and emotional signs. Here are some common indicators that your child may be experiencing gut-related problems:

- **Digestive Symptoms:** Bloating, gas, constipation, diarrhea, or stomach pain are the most obvious signs of gut issues.
- **Food Sensitivities:** Children with imbalanced gut flora are often more prone to food sensitivities, reacting negatively to common foods like gluten, dairy, or processed sugars.
- **Behavioral Changes:** Mood swings, irritability, difficulty concentrating, or hyperactivity can sometimes be traced back to poor gut health.
- **Skin Issues:** Eczema, rashes, and other skin conditions may

be linked to gut health, as the skin often reflects internal imbalances.

Understanding these signs is crucial in identifying when your child's gut may need extra support. By addressing digestive health early, you can prevent larger issues from arising down the road.

Healing and Supporting Gut Health

Foods and Supplements for a Healthy Gut

The good news is that gut health can be supported and healed naturally through diet and targeted supplements. Here are some of the best ways to nourish the gut:

- **Probiotics:** These beneficial bacteria can help restore balance in the gut, crowding out harmful bacteria and supporting overall gut function. Foods like yogurt, kefir, and fermented vegetables (like sauerkraut and kimchi) are rich in probiotics. Supplements can also be an effective way to ensure your child is getting enough probiotics, especially if they are dealing with digestive issues.
- **Prebiotics:** Prebiotics are the food for good bacteria, helping them thrive in the gut. Foods rich in fiber, like bananas, onions, garlic, and asparagus, are excellent sources of prebiotics.
- **Fermented Foods:** Fermented foods are packed with beneficial bacteria that help restore the gut's balance. Examples include miso, kombucha, and tempeh.
- **Whole, Unprocessed Foods:** A diet rich in vegetables, fruits, whole grains, and lean proteins supports gut health by providing essential nutrients that nourish both the body and the gut microbiome.

- **Bone Broth:** This healing food is rich in collagen and amino acids that support the gut lining, making it especially helpful for children with digestive issues like leaky gut.

Holistic Remedies for Gut Issues

If your child is experiencing gut-related discomfort, there are gentle, natural remedies that can help restore balance without resorting to harsh medications. These holistic options support digestion, relieve bloating, and promote a healthy gut environment.

1. **Herbal Teas**

- **Chamomile, Ginger, and Peppermint Teas**: These teas are gentle yet effective for soothing digestive discomfort, reducing bloating, and calming the nervous system. Chamomile is particularly helpful for relaxation, ginger can reduce nausea, and peppermint eases gas and stomach cramps.

2. **Probiotics**

- **Gut Health Support**: Probiotics introduce beneficial bacteria into the gut, which helps balance the microbiome. Look for strains like *Lactobacillus* and *Bifidobacterium*, which are safe for children and promote digestive health, reduce gas, and support immune function.
- **Daily Use**: Probiotics can be found in foods like yogurt, kefir, and certain fermented foods, or as supplements specifically formulated for kids.

3. **Digestive Enzymes**

- **Aid for Digestion**: Digestive enzymes can help children break down food more efficiently, especially if they struggle with food sensitivities or indigestion. Enzymes like amylase, lipase, and protease make nutrients easier to absorb, reducing digestive strain and discomfort.
- **When to Use**: These enzymes are often taken before meals to support digestion, especially when introducing new foods or foods that may cause sensitivities.

4. Activated Charcoal

- **Detoxifying Aid**: Activated charcoal binds to toxins and gas-producing compounds in the digestive tract, which can alleviate bloating and gas. It's especially useful for acute digestive discomfort but should only be used occasionally, as it can also absorb nutrients if overused.
- **Safe Practices**: Always consult a pediatrician before using activated charcoal with young children, and avoid using it alongside medications, as it can reduce their effectiveness.

5. Slippery Elm and Marshmallow Root

- **Soothing the Gut Lining**: These mucilaginous herbs create a protective coating on the gut lining, which helps reduce inflammation and provides relief for conditions like leaky gut or IBS. Slippery elm and marshmallow root are often used in tea or powder form.
- **Gentle Relief**: Both herbs are known for their ability to soothe irritation, making them excellent for sensitive digestive systems.

6. Fennel

- **Gas and Bloating Relief**: Fennel has natural anti-spasmodic properties that help relax the muscles in the gastrointestinal tract, reducing gas and bloating. Fennel seeds or fennel tea can be especially useful after meals to relieve discomfort.
- **Gentle on the Stomach**: Fennel is mild enough for children and can be consumed in tea or added to food for a hint of flavor while promoting digestive comfort.

Supporting Gut Health Naturally

Incorporating these remedies into your child's routine provides gentle support for their digestive health. By addressing gut issues naturally, you help maintain a balanced microbiome, reduce digestive discomfort, and support overall well-being. Remember to consult with a healthcare provider before introducing any new remedies, especially with young children, to ensure safe and effective use.

Transitioning to Solids: Supporting Gut Health from the Start

The transition from breastmilk or formula to solid foods is a key milestone in a child's development, especially for their digestive health. A thoughtful approach to introducing solids can support healthy gut flora, reduce the likelihood of sensitivities, and encourage a well-rounded palate. Whether you choose purees, baby-led weaning, or a combination of both, a gradual transition helps the digestive system adapt and flourish.

When to Start Solids

- **Ideal Timing**: The American Academy of Pediatrics generally recommends starting solids around **6 months** when babies show readiness cues, such as sitting up with support, showing interest in food, and losing the tongue-thrust reflex (pushing objects out of the mouth).
- **Why Timing Matters for Gut Health**: At 6 months, the digestive system has typically developed enough to handle new foods. Starting solids too early can stress a baby's digestive system, leading to potential food sensitivities and an imbalance in gut bacteria.

Baby-Led Weaning vs. Purees

- **Baby-Led Weaning (BLW)**: This approach encourages babies to self-feed soft, manageable pieces of food instead of spoon-fed purees. BLW can foster independence and help babies develop their chewing skills and motor coordination.
- **BLW and Gut Health**: Allowing babies to chew and experience different textures can stimulate enzyme production in the digestive tract, which aids in breaking down foods efficiently and supports gut health.
- **Purees**: Spoon-fed purees can be an ideal way to start solids, especially if there are concerns about choking or if babies need extra help in transitioning to more solid textures. Purees provide easily digestible nutrients that are gentle on the developing gut.
- **Combination Approach**: Some parents find success in combining both methods. Offering purees alongside manageable finger foods lets babies explore a variety of tastes and textures.

Introducing Foods Gradually

- **Simple, Whole Foods**: Start with single-ingredient foods like cooked vegetables (carrots, sweet potatoes), soft fruits (bananas, avocados), and iron-rich options (like well-cooked lentils or soft-cooked egg yolk).
- **One at a Time**: Introduce one new food every 3-5 days to monitor for potential sensitivities. This gradual approach also allows the gut microbiome to adjust slowly, supporting its stability and resilience.
- **Iron-Rich Foods**: Around 6 months, babies' iron stores begin to diminish, so incorporating iron-rich foods (such as fortified cereals, lentils, and meats) helps replenish these levels and supports gut and overall health.

Foods to Avoid in the First Year

- **Honey**: Avoid honey entirely until after the first year, as it can contain spores of *Clostridium botulinum*, which can lead to infant botulism due to babies' immature digestive systems.
- **Whole Nuts and Large Chunks**: Nuts and large chunks of hard foods can pose a choking hazard. Instead, opt for nut butters thinned with water or milk or very small pieces of soft foods.
- **Cow's Milk as a Primary Drink**: Although dairy can be introduced in small amounts (like yogurt or cheese), cow's milk shouldn't be a primary drink until after age one, as it can be difficult to digest and may lead to iron deficiency.
- **Highly Processed and Sugary Foods**: Avoid added sugars and highly processed foods to prevent disrupting the natural

gut bacteria balance. Early exposure to these foods can promote an unhealthy microbiome.

- **Limit Acidic and Salty Foods**: High salt and acidic foods (like citrus in large amounts) can be too harsh on a baby's developing gut lining.

Timing and Progression of Food Introductions

- **6-8 Months**: Begin with soft fruits, vegetables, whole grains, and purees or manageable finger foods. Focus on easy-to-digest foods that are nutrient-dense and low in potential allergens.
- **8-10 Months**: Add more variety, including lean proteins, legumes, and small amounts of dairy (like yogurt and cheese). This period is also ideal for introducing more textures, which stimulate digestive enzyme production and enhance gut function.
- **10-12 Months**: Babies can handle more complex food combinations and a wider variety of textures, including soft-cooked meats, mixed dishes, and a broader range of fruits and vegetables.

Supporting Gut Health During Transition

- **Encourage Probiotic-Rich Foods**: Introducing yogurt or kefir after 8 months can provide beneficial bacteria to support gut flora. Probiotics play a critical role in maintaining a healthy balance in the digestive system, which is important for immunity and digestion.
- **Include Fiber-Rich Foods**: Fruits, vegetables, and whole grains contain fiber, which supports the growth of healthy

gut bacteria. Fiber acts as prebiotics, feeding beneficial bacteria in the gut and promoting a balanced microbiome.

- **Watch for Signs of Sensitivity**: Gas, rashes, or digestive upset could indicate that a food is hard for your baby to digest. If a reaction occurs, pause that food and discuss with your pediatrician before reintroducing it.

The Gut Health Connection

A gentle, gradual introduction to solids can be incredibly beneficial for a baby's digestive system. By slowly exposing the gut to different foods, parents help build a robust, healthy microbiome, which can reduce the likelihood of digestive issues, food sensitivities, and infections. A balanced approach to starting solids—whether through baby-led weaning, purees, or a mix of both—supports not only physical development but also long-term digestive health, creating a foundation for wellness in childhood and beyond.

Probiotics for Infants After C-Section: Supporting Gut Health Early

Infants born via C-section may have different gut bacteria than those born vaginally, as they miss the exposure to beneficial bacteria from the birth canal. Introducing probiotics can support gut colonization and potentially improve digestion, immunity, and long-term health outcomes.

Why C-Section Birth Affects the Gut Microbiome

- **Differences in Bacteria**: Vaginal birth provides infants with beneficial bacteria from the mother's microbiome, helping to "seed" or establish healthy gut bacteria early on. C-section births bypass this exposure, leading to a different gut bacteria composition, often with fewer beneficial strains.

- **Potential Health Implications**: Research suggests that C-section babies are at higher risk for conditions like allergies, asthma, and obesity, potentially due to differences in their early microbiome. Supporting gut health with probiotics may help mitigate some of these risks.

Introducing Probiotics for Infants

- **Choosing a Probiotic**: Look for probiotics formulated specifically for infants, containing strains such as *Bifidobacterium* and *Lactobacillus*, which are gentle and support a healthy gut.
- **Methods of Administration**: Probiotics can be given as drops, added to breastmilk, or mixed with formula. Always follow the dosage instructions and consult a pediatrician before introducing any supplement.
- **Benefits for Gut Health**: Early probiotic supplementation may support immune function, digestion, and nutrient absorption by promoting a balanced microbiome. This can be especially beneficial for C-section babies, helping them develop a microbiome similar to that of vaginally delivered infants.

Connecting Probiotics to Lifelong Gut Health

Establishing a healthy microbiome early in life is critical for long-term gut health. Introducing probiotics after a C-section can aid in developing a resilient digestive system, support immune function, and reduce the likelihood of digestive and immune-related issues as the child grows.

Understanding the Bristol Stool Chart for Children's Gut Health

The Bristol Stool Chart is a useful tool for assessing digestive health by examining the shape and consistency of stool. For parents, understanding where their child's bowel movements fall on the chart can help identify possible digestive issues and indicate what changes may be needed in their diet or health regimen.

Stool Types and Nutritional Adjustments:

Type 1 (Separate Hard Lumps): Indicates constipation. Increase water intake and add more fiber-rich foods such as fruits, vegetables, and whole grains.

Type 2 (Lumpy and Sausage-Like): Suggests mild constipation. Encourage more fluids and foods that promote bowel regularity, like prunes or chia seeds.

Type 3 (Sausage Shape with Cracks): Normal but could benefit from more hydration.

Type 4 (Smooth, Soft Sausage): Ideal and indicates healthy digestion.

Type 5 (Soft Blobs with Clear-Cut Edges): May indicate a lack of fiber. Include more complex carbohydrates and high-fiber snacks.

Type 6 (Mushy with Ragged Edges): Can indicate mild diarrhea. Reduce sugar intake and consider foods like bananas and rice.

Type 7 (Entirely Liquid): Points to severe diarrhea. Ensure hydration and consider probiotics to restore gut flora.

By understanding the Bristol Stool Chart and making dietary adjustments based on its insights, parents can support their child's digestive health and foster a balanced gut environment.

The Hidden Dangers of Food Coloring and Industry Oversight

Artificial food colorings are prevalent in many processed foods, especially those aimed at children, such as candies, cereals, and snacks. Despite their bright appeal, many food dyes are associated with health risks, particularly for the gut and brain. Inadequate regulation within the food industry means these additives often make their way into products with little transparency or warning about their potential effects on children's health.

1. **What Are Artificial Food Dyes?**

- **Types of Common Dyes**: Artificial food colorings like Red 40, Yellow 5, and Blue 1 are petroleum-based chemicals designed to enhance the color and appeal of processed foods. These dyes are prevalent in snacks, sugary drinks, cereals, and even products marketed as "healthy."
- **Lack of Stringent Regulation**: The U.S. FDA allows many synthetic dyes in the food supply, but regulation is minimal. While some European countries require warning labels on foods with artificial dyes or have banned certain colorants, the U.S. does not have the same strict regulations.

2. Neurotoxic Effects of Food Dyes

- **Impact on Behavior and Attention**: Research indicates that artificial food dyes may contribute to hyperactivity, attention issues, and behavioral changes in children, particularly those with ADHD. These dyes can disrupt neurotransmitter function and brain health, which in turn affects mood and behavior.
- **Neurotoxicity and Learning**: Neurotoxic compounds in food dyes may impair cognitive development. For growing brains, repeated exposure to these chemicals can lead to challenges in learning, impulse control, and social behavior, making them especially concerning for young children.

3. Disrupting Gut Health

- **Gut-Brain Connection**: The gut and brain communicate through what's known as the gut-brain axis. Artificial dyes can disrupt this balance by altering gut bacteria and damaging the gut lining, which can lead to inflammation and a weakened microbiome.

- **Impact on Microbiome Balance**: Synthetic dyes can act as irritants to gut cells, promoting inflammation and allowing harmful bacteria to thrive. This disruption can lead to symptoms like bloating, constipation, or diarrhea and may contribute to immune issues over time.

4. Choosing Natural Alternatives

- **Natural Color Sources**: Bright colors from natural sources, like turmeric (yellow), beet juice (red), and spirulina (blue-green), can be safer alternatives. Look for products labeled with natural colorants or choose whole foods, which don't rely on artificial enhancement.
- **Reading Labels**: To avoid artificial dyes, check ingredient labels carefully. Terms like "Red 40," "Yellow 5," or "FD&C" indicate synthetic dyes, whereas natural colors are usually listed by their source, such as "beet juice" or "turmeric."

A Healthier Approach to Food Choices

Reducing artificial food dyes in children's diets can make a significant difference in their gut health, behavior, and overall development. By opting for naturally colored foods and becoming aware of the limited regulation surrounding food additives, parents can help protect their children's gut microbiome and support more balanced mood and behavior. This approach supports both digestive and neurological health, offering a simple yet impactful way to safeguard against common environmental toxins.

Raw vs. Pasteurized Milk: Weighing the Pros and Cons

Milk is a staple in many diets, but choosing between raw and pasteurized milk has become a topic of debate. Both types offer potential benefits, but they also come with risks that may affect gut health and overall wellness.

Raw Milk

- **Pros**:
- **Rich in Enzymes and Beneficial Bacteria**: Raw milk is unpasteurized, preserving naturally occurring enzymes and probiotics. These beneficial bacteria can support gut health, strengthen the immune system, and aid digestion.
- **Nutrient Density**: Many raw milk advocates believe it retains more vitamins, minerals, and fats than pasteurized milk, which may contribute to better nutrient absorption.
- **Cons**:
- **Risk of Contamination**: Since raw milk is not heated to kill bacteria, it can carry harmful pathogens like *E. coli*, *Salmonella*, and *Listeria*. For young children, pregnant women, and immunocompromised individuals, this risk is especially concerning.
- **Regulation and Accessibility**: Raw milk is illegal in some states due to safety concerns, and sourcing high-quality, safe raw milk can be challenging.

Pasteurized Milk

- **Pros**:
- **Enhanced Safety**: Pasteurization heats milk to eliminate harmful bacteria, significantly reducing the risk of food-

borne illness.

- **Longer Shelf Life**: Pasteurized milk has a longer shelf life than raw milk, making it more convenient and accessible for many families.
- **Cons**:
- **Loss of Enzymes and Bacteria**: The pasteurization process kills both harmful and beneficial bacteria, which may reduce the potential gut health benefits found in raw milk.
- **Potential for Reduced Nutrients**: Heating milk may diminish some vitamins, minerals, and enzymes, which could impact its nutritional value.

In summary, raw milk offers probiotic benefits for the gut but carries health risks due to potential bacterial contamination. Pasteurized milk provides a safer option but lacks the probiotic benefits that raw milk can offer for digestive health.

GMOs, Artificial Sweeteners, and High-Fructose Corn Syrup: Gut Disruptors

Genetically modified organisms (GMOs), artificial sweeteners, and high-fructose corn syrup (HFCS) are common additives in processed foods. While these ingredients increase convenience and flavor, they can also disrupt gut health and impact overall wellness.

1. **GMOs (Genetically Modified Organisms)**

- **What Are GMOs?**: GMOs are plants or animals genetically altered for improved yield, resistance to pests, or other qualities. Crops like corn and soy are commonly modified, and products containing these ingredients are often processed and refined.

- **Impact on Gut Health**: Some studies suggest that GMOs may alter gut bacteria balance and lead to inflammation in the digestive tract. Pesticides used in GMO farming, like glyphosate, can negatively affect gut bacteria diversity and integrity.

2. Artificial Sweeteners

- **Types of Artificial Sweeteners**: Common artificial sweeteners include aspartame, sucralose, and saccharin. These are frequently found in "sugar-free" or "diet" products.
- **Impact on Gut Health**: Artificial sweeteners are not absorbed in the same way as natural sugars and can disturb gut flora by feeding harmful bacteria. Studies have linked artificial sweeteners to imbalances in gut bacteria, potentially leading to digestive discomfort and metabolic issues.

3. High-Fructose Corn Syrup (HFCS)

- **What Is HFCS?**: HFCS is a highly processed sweetener made from corn starch. Found in sodas, baked goods, and condiments, it's known for its affordability and sweetness.
- **Impact on Gut Health**: HFCS is metabolized differently than natural sugars, leading to excessive fructose in the gut, which can disrupt the microbiome. High intake of HFCS is associated with increased inflammation, leaky gut, and higher risks of metabolic diseases.

The Gut Health Connection

These additives are prevalent in processed foods, but their effects on the gut should not be underestimated. GMOs, artificial sweeteners, and HFCS can contribute to inflammation, alter gut bacteria, and increase the risk of digestive issues. For a healthier gut and more balanced microbiome, minimizing processed foods and choosing whole, organic foods whenever possible can support digestive wellness and reduce exposure to these potentially harmful additives.

Holistic Remedies for Gut Issues and the Gut's Role in Emotional Health

If your child is experiencing gut-related discomfort, there are gentle, natural remedies that can help restore balance without resorting to harsh medications. Supporting gut health is not only beneficial for digestion but also plays a crucial role in emotional well-being, as the gut produces neurotransmitters like serotonin and dopamine, which influence mood, focus, and behavior. Additionally, the gut releases GLP-1 (glucagon-like peptide-1), a hormone that aids in regulating blood sugar and appetite.

1. **Neurotransmitters in the Gut**

- **Serotonin**: Often called the "feel-good" neurotransmitter, serotonin helps regulate mood, sleep, and appetite. Remarkably, around 90% of the body's serotonin is produced in the gut, meaning that a balanced gut environment supports better emotional health and reduces symptoms like anxiety and irritability.

- **Dopamine**: Known for its role in motivation, reward, and focus, dopamine is partially synthesized in the gut. A healthy gut microbiome supports dopamine production, contributing to improved concentration and emotional stability in children.

2. **GLP-1 (Glucagon-Like Peptide-1)**

- **Role in Blood Sugar Regulation and Appetite Control**: GLP-1 is a hormone produced in the gut that helps regulate blood sugar levels by enhancing insulin secretion and slowing digestion. It also contributes to feelings of satiety, helping children develop a healthy relationship with food.
- **Gut Health Impact**: An imbalanced microbiome can affect GLP-1 production, potentially influencing blood sugar regulation and appetite control. Supporting a healthy gut environment aids in stabilizing GLP-1 production, which can be especially helpful for children's overall metabolic health.

Holistic Remedies for Gut Health

These holistic remedies not only aid in relieving digestive discomfort but also support the gut's vital role in producing neurotransmitters and hormones that impact mental and metabolic health.

3. **Herbal Teas**

- **Chamomile, Ginger, and Peppermint Teas**: These teas are gentle yet effective for soothing digestive discomfort, reducing bloating, and calming the nervous system. Chamomile promotes relaxation, ginger eases nausea, and peppermint reduces gas and stomach cramps.

4. Probiotics

- **Gut Health Support**: Probiotics introduce beneficial bacteria into the gut, balancing the microbiome. Strains like *Lactobacillus* and *Bifidobacterium* support digestion, reduce gas, and promote serotonin production, enhancing mood and emotional well-being.
- **Daily Use**: Probiotics are found in yogurt, kefir, and fermented foods or as supplements for kids, supporting both digestive health and neurotransmitter production.

5. Digestive Enzymes

- **Aid for Digestion**: Digestive enzymes help break down food more efficiently, which can benefit children with food sensitivities or indigestion. By aiding nutrient absorption, enzymes contribute to a healthy gut environment that supports neurotransmitter production.

6. Activated Charcoal

- **Detoxifying Aid**: Activated charcoal binds to toxins in the digestive tract, reducing gas and bloating. Use this occasionally for acute discomfort, but consult a pediatrician before giving it to children to avoid nutrient absorption issues.

7. Slippery Elm and Marshmallow Root

- **Soothing the Gut Lining**: These mucilaginous herbs coat the gut lining, reducing inflammation and relieving discomfort. A healthy gut lining supports efficient neurotransmitter and GLP-1 production, which are essential for emotional regulation and metabolic stability.

8. Fennel

- **Gas and Bloating Relief**: Fennel relaxes the gastrointestinal tract, reducing gas and promoting gut health. It's mild enough for children, with the added benefit of enhancing the gut's ability to produce essential neurotransmitters.

Supporting Gut Health Naturally

By incorporating these remedies into your child's routine, you support not only their digestive health but also the production of key neurotransmitters and hormones. A balanced gut contributes to improved emotional well-being, reduced behavioral issues, and better metabolic health, showing just how integral gut health is to your child's overall wellness. Remember to consult with a healthcare provider before introducing new remedies to ensure safe and effective use.

A Family's Transformation through a Gut-Healing Diet

The Jackson family's story is a powerful example of how a gut-healing diet can transform a child's health. Their son, Dylan, had struggled with eczema and ADHD symptoms for years. After numerous doctor visits and a reliance on medications that seemed to only provide temporary relief, the family decided to take a different approach. They worked with a holistic health practitioner to identify food sensitivities and began incorporating a gut-healing diet rich in probiotics, prebiotics, and nutrient-dense whole foods. Within months, Dylan's eczema cleared up, his attention span improved, and his behavioral issues became more manageable. The family was amazed at how much better he felt once his gut was restored to balance.

Children's Quirky Reactions to Fermented Foods

Introducing fermented foods to kids can be an adventure in itself. One mother recalls the first time she gave her daughter a taste of kombucha—a fermented tea full of probiotics. Her daughter's face scrunched up in confusion and amusement as she declared, "It's fizzy, sour, and kind of weird, but I like it!" Similarly, when another family introduced sauerkraut to their children, the kids were hesitant at first, but after trying it, they began to request "the crunchy cabbage" with their meals. These small steps toward gut health often come with fun and surprising reactions from kids who are learning to appreciate new flavors and textures.

A healthy gut is pivotal to a child's overall wellness, influencing not only physical health but also emotional balance and cognitive development. By paying attention to gut health and supporting it with the right foods and natural remedies, you are giving your child a solid foundation for long-term health.

This chapter emphasizes the importance of seeing food as medicine. By focusing on gut health, you're reinforcing the broader commitment to natural health practices, which are central to the crunchy lifestyle. Supporting the gut means supporting the whole child—physically, emotionally, and mentally.

In the next chapter, we'll explore how to nurture your child's natural growth and development without unnecessary interventions. We'll discuss the importance of trusting your child's developmental timeline and encouraging creativity and play as essential elements of a balanced life.

8

Nurturing Natural Growth and Development

Consider the miracle of natural growth—how a tiny seed transforms into a towering tree over time, given the right environment and care. Like nature, children grow and develop in their own unique ways and at their own pace. Each stage of development requires thoughtful support, not intervention. Rushing the process can often do more harm than good. As parents, we must learn to trust that, given the right conditions, our children will flourish naturally. This chapter explores how supporting your child's growth through holistic practices can create a solid foundation for lifelong wellness.

Supporting your child's natural growth through holistic practices fosters resilience, creativity, and emotional well-being. Rather than focusing on hitting milestones by a certain age or overloading children with structured activities, the goal is to nurture their innate curiosity, encourage play, and provide an environment where they can grow at their own pace. By trusting in your child's unique developmental timeline, you allow them to reach their full potential without unnecessary pressure.

Trusting Natural Milestones

Avoiding Over-Scheduling

In today's fast-paced world, parents often feel pressure to enroll their children in numerous activities, from sports to music lessons, in hopes of giving them a competitive edge. However, over-scheduling can stifle a child's natural curiosity and creativity. Free time—time to simply play, imagine, and explore the world at their own pace—is essential for healthy development.

When children are given the freedom to engage in unstructured play, they learn to solve problems, express emotions, and explore their interests on their own terms. This kind of play fosters resilience, as children learn to navigate challenges without the constant direction of adults. It also encourages creativity, which is essential for intellectual and emotional growth.

As parents, we must resist the urge to fill every moment of our child's day with structured activities. Instead, let them play freely, whether that's building a fort in the backyard, drawing, or simply daydreaming. These moments of unstructured play are when children often discover their passions and develop skills that will serve them throughout life.

Developmental Milestones

Every child grows and develops at their own pace, and while developmental milestones can be helpful guides, they are not set in stone. Some children may start walking or talking earlier than others, while some may take a bit more time to master certain skills. Trusting your child's unique growth timeline is key to fostering their confidence and well-being.

It's important to remember that milestones are not deadlines. Rushing your child into activities or therapies before they are ready can create unnecessary stress and anxiety. Instead, observe your child's natural inclinations and offer gentle support as they progress through each stage of development. Celebrate their achievements, no matter when they occur, and trust that they will reach each milestone in their own time.

Supporting Mental Growth

Creativity and Play

Creativity is a powerful force in child development. Through play, children explore new ideas, solve problems, and express emotions. Unstructured playtime allows children to use their imagination, experiment with different roles, and make sense of the world around them. Whether they're building imaginary worlds with toys or inventing games with friends, creativity is a cornerstone of intellectual and emotional development.

Allowing children to explore their creative side without rigid boundaries helps them become confident in their ability to think independently and approach challenges with an open mind. Encouraging play and exploration also builds emotional resilience, as children learn to navigate both success and failure in a safe and nurturing environment.

Holistic Learning Environments

Creating spaces and experiences that foster curiosity is another essential part of supporting your child's mental growth. A holistic learning environment doesn't rely on formal instruction alone—it's about providing your child with opportunities to explore the world in meaningful ways. This can include everything from nature walks to hands-on activities like cooking, gardening, or building.

At home, create spaces where your child feels free to explore their interests, whether it's a quiet corner for reading, an art station stocked with supplies, or access to puzzles and building blocks that encourage problem-solving. Engaging with the natural world is also a powerful way to foster curiosity. Outdoor play, whether in a backyard or a local park, offers countless opportunities for discovery and learning.

By focusing on experiences that stimulate curiosity and creativity, you help your child develop a love of learning that will last a lifetime.

Theories on Child Development: Foundations and Insights for Natural Parenting

Child development theories offer valuable insights into how children grow, learn, and adapt to their environment. For parents embracing a "crunchy" or holistic approach, understanding these theories can help create supportive environments that align with natural health practices, respect for individual growth, and a nurturing of both physical and emotional well-being. Here are some influential theories and their potential applications for natural parenting.

1. **Jean Piaget's Cognitive Development Theory**

- **Who Was Piaget?** Jean Piaget was a Swiss psychologist known for his work in child development. He proposed that children progress through four stages of cognitive development, each marked by unique abilities and ways of understanding the world: Sensorimotor, Preoperational, Concrete Operational, and Formal Operational.
- **Core Concept**: Piaget believed that children are active learners who construct knowledge through their interactions with the environment. He emphasized the importance of exploration, hands-on activities, and self-directed learn-

ing.

- **Crunchy Mom Takeaway**: Encouraging open-ended play, nature exploration, and independent learning opportunities aligns well with Piaget's theory. By allowing children to explore and discover at their own pace, we respect their individual development stages and promote cognitive growth without the need for formalized, rigid instruction.

2. Lev Vygotsky's Sociocultural Theory

- **Who Was Vygotsky?** Lev Vygotsky was a Russian psychologist who emphasized the social and cultural aspects of learning. His theory suggests that children learn through social interactions and that adults play a crucial role by providing guidance and support within the child's "Zone of Proximal Development" (ZPD).
- **Core Concept**: Vygotsky's theory highlights the importance of community, social interactions, and cultural influences on a child's cognitive development. He argued that learning is collaborative and happens best when adults scaffold or support children as they learn new skills.
- **Crunchy Mom Takeaway**: Vygotsky's ideas reinforce the value of community-based learning, like homeschool co-ops and family involvement. Encouraging family participation in daily tasks, engaging with different age groups, and allowing children to learn through social settings fosters growth and learning. It also highlights the importance of role-modeling healthy behaviors, values, and practices for children.

3. Maria Montessori's Montessori Method

- **Who Was Montessori?** Maria Montessori was an Italian physician and educator who developed the Montessori Method, a child-centered approach to education based on self-directed activity, hands-on learning, and collaborative play.
- **Core Concept**: The Montessori Method encourages children to learn at their own pace in a prepared environment. It focuses on building independence, encouraging exploration, and fostering intrinsic motivation.
- **Crunchy Mom Takeaway**: Montessori's approach aligns well with a natural parenting perspective. Creating a child-friendly home environment where children have accessible, natural materials fosters independence and encourages exploration. This method promotes the use of real-world activities, such as cooking or gardening, that children can engage in alongside adults. Montessori also advocates for minimal plastic toys, favoring natural, wooden materials—something many crunchy moms appreciate for reducing exposure to harmful chemicals.

4. Erik Erikson's Psychosocial Development Theory

- **Who Was Erikson?** Erik Erikson was a developmental psychologist who proposed that people go through eight stages of psychosocial development, each marked by a central conflict. His theory focuses on the development of identity and the importance of social relationships.
- **Core Concept**: Erikson's stages outline key psychosocial challenges, such as trust vs. mistrust and autonomy vs. shame, that children must navigate as they grow. He emphasized the importance of supportive and nurturing

relationships for healthy development.

- **Crunchy Mom Takeaway**: Erikson's theory reinforces the need for a secure, loving environment where children feel safe to explore and develop autonomy. Practicing attachment parenting, such as baby-wearing, breastfeeding, and responsive caregiving, supports Erikson's focus on building trust and fostering emotional resilience. Crunchy moms can take Erikson's insights as a reminder to offer children opportunities for independence while also providing a stable, comforting presence.

5. Rudolf Steiner's Waldorf Education Theory

- **Who Was Steiner?** Rudolf Steiner was an Austrian philosopher who developed the Waldorf approach, which views education as a holistic process that integrates intellectual, artistic, and practical skills.
- **Core Concept**: Waldorf education emphasizes the rhythm of daily life, creative play, and imagination, promoting learning through natural experiences rather than through rote memorization or testing. Steiner believed in protecting children's natural sense of wonder by delaying formal academics and focusing on play and creativity in early childhood.
- **Crunchy Mom Takeaway**: The Waldorf approach aligns well with holistic parenting values, as it emphasizes the use of natural materials, limited screen time, and a strong connection to nature. For parents, incorporating Waldorf-inspired practices might include establishing family rituals, using seasonal activities, and providing open-ended, natural toys. Steiner's approach also reinforces the importance

of a stress-free environment, where children are shielded from external pressures.

6. John Bowlby's Attachment Theory

- **Who Was Bowlby?** John Bowlby was a British psychologist known for his work in attachment theory, which focuses on the importance of secure attachments between children and their caregivers.
- **Core Concept**: Bowlby's theory suggests that a secure attachment provides a foundation for healthy emotional and social development. Children who feel secure in their attachment to caregivers are more likely to explore, take risks, and develop resilience.
- **Crunchy Mom Takeaway**: Attachment parenting practices, such as co-sleeping, breastfeeding, and being responsive to children's needs, are central to this theory. A "crunchy mom" might prioritize creating a nurturing, consistent environment to build secure attachments. This aligns with the belief that a strong emotional foundation supports lifelong well-being, independence, and confidence.

7. Howard Gardner's Multiple Intelligences Theory

- **Who Was Gardner?** Howard Gardner is a developmental psychologist who proposed the theory of multiple intelligences, which suggests that intelligence is not a single general ability but rather a range of distinct types, such as linguistic, logical-mathematical, spatial, and kinesthetic intelligence.
- **Core Concept**: Gardner's theory emphasizes the diversity

of human potential and the importance of recognizing each child's unique strengths. He argues that traditional schooling often overlooks non-academic talents, which are just as valuable.

- **Crunchy Mom Takeaway**: Gardner's ideas support a child-led approach to learning, recognizing each child's strengths rather than a one-size-fits-all model. For crunchy parents, this could mean offering diverse activities like music, art, outdoor exploration, and hands-on tasks, allowing children to explore a range of interests. It reinforces the idea that there's no single pathway to learning, and embracing individuality can foster a more enriching environment for children.

8. Lawrence Kohlberg's Moral Development Theory

- **Who Was Kohlberg?** Lawrence Kohlberg was a psychologist known for his theory of moral development, which describes how children develop an understanding of morality through stages of moral reasoning.
- **Core Concept**: Kohlberg suggested that children progress from understanding right and wrong based on punishment and reward to higher stages where they recognize universal ethical principles. Moral development, according to Kohlberg, is a gradual process influenced by experiences and social interactions.
- **Crunchy Mom Takeaway**: Kohlberg's theory reminds parents that children need space and time to explore ethical questions and learn empathy. Modeling empathy, respect for nature, and kindness within the family can nurture children's moral development. Activities like helping with

family chores, volunteering, or discussing the impact of personal choices (e.g., Eco-friendly practices) can help children internalize values rather than simply following rules.

Final Thoughts: Honoring Your Child's Unique Journey

Each of these child development theories provides a valuable lens through which to view your child's growth and learning. By taking a "crunchy mom" approach, you can apply these insights holistically, creating a supportive environment that respects your child's unique needs, fosters natural growth, and emphasizes a strong, nurturing connection. The key is to trust in your child's individual path and recognize that development is a deeply personal process, best nurtured by patience, openness, and a balanced approach to learning and life.

Choosing the Best Educational Path for Your Child: Finding What Works for Your Family

The choice of schooling or childcare can feel overwhelming, with so many options and considerations to balance. From daycare to homeschool, and from public schools to specialized environments like Montessori, the decision often brings societal pressures, expectations, and opinions. Ultimately, it's essential to prioritize your child's unique needs and your family's values, lifestyle, and comfort.

Understanding Different Educational Options

1. **Daycare and Early Childhood Programs**

- **Benefits**: Many daycare and early childhood programs provide a structured environment for young children, supporting socialization, motor skills, and foundational learning. Quality programs also help children develop routines, share, and interact with peers.
- **Considerations**: Look into each daycare's curriculum, caregiver-to-child ratio, and staff qualifications. For families who need consistent childcare, daycare provides a dependable schedule, but it's crucial to feel comfortable with the environment and caregivers.

1. **Homeschooling**

- **Benefits**: Homeschooling offers flexibility in curriculum, teaching methods, and daily schedule, allowing parents to tailor education to each child's pace and interests. Families often choose homeschooling to focus on specific values, interests, or health needs.
- **Considerations**: Homeschooling requires a significant commitment of time and resources from parents or guardians, and it's beneficial to connect with local homeschooling communities or online groups for support. Families should assess whether they have the time, patience, and resources to make homeschooling work for their lifestyle.

1. **Homeschool Co-Ops**

- **Benefits**: Homeschool co-ops combine the benefits of homeschooling with group learning. These co-ops typically gather several families together for shared lessons, field trips, or activities, providing socialization and specialized group classes that parents may not feel equipped to teach alone.

- **Considerations**: Co-ops vary in structure; some meet weekly while others meet several times a month. They can offer great resources and community, but they still require a commitment from parents in terms of teaching or assisting. Look for a co-op that aligns with your educational goals, teaching philosophies, and schedule.

1. **Church Schools**

- **Benefits**: Church-based schools offer an environment that emphasizes faith and community values, often with smaller class sizes and a supportive atmosphere. They provide structured learning with a curriculum that may align with family values.
- **Considerations**: Families should ensure that the curriculum aligns with their beliefs and educational expectations. Church schools can be more affordable than private schools but may lack specialized programs found in larger institutions.

1. **Public Schools**

- **Benefits**: Public schools offer a variety of resources, such as sports teams, extracurricular activities, and specialized classes. They follow a standardized curriculum and provide a setting where children can learn to navigate diverse social environments.
- **Considerations**: Public schools have larger class sizes and varied funding, which may affect the quality of education.

Families should evaluate local schools to determine whether they offer the support, resources, and culture they want for their children. For many families, public schools provide a balanced option in terms of accessibility and structure.

1. **Private Schools**

- **Benefits**: Private schools often provide smaller class sizes, specialized curricula, and additional resources for individualized learning. Many private schools offer advanced programs, a range of extracurricular activities, and a focused approach to academics or the arts.
- **Considerations**: Private schools typically require tuition and may have rigorous admission requirements. It's essential to research whether the school's educational philosophy and culture match what you envision for your child.

1. **Montessori Schools**

- **Benefits**: Montessori schools focus on child-led, hands-on learning, fostering independence and critical thinking. Classrooms are typically multi-age, allowing children to learn at their own pace and interact with peers of various ages.
- **Considerations**: The Montessori approach may not be for everyone, especially if a child requires more structure or has difficulty adapting to a self-paced environment. Montessori schools can be costly, and families should observe classrooms to see if this method fits their child's learning style and personality.

Key Factors to Consider for Each Option

Regardless of the setting, here are some essential factors to weigh when choosing a school or educational path:

1. **Learning Style and Personality**: Each child learns differently—some thrive in hands-on, self-directed environments, while others prefer structured, teacher-led instruction. Considering your child's unique personality and how they respond to different learning styles can help you choose a program that makes them feel engaged and comfortable.
2. **Family Lifestyle and Schedule**: Certain educational choices require a considerable time investment from parents (like homeschooling or co-ops), while others provide a more flexible schedule (like daycare or public school). Your family's work schedule, commitments, and lifestyle can significantly influence what works best.
3. **Values and Educational Goals**: Many families prioritize education that aligns with their values, whether that's faith-based learning, progressive education, or a focus on the arts. Clarifying what you want from an educational experience can help you navigate the options with a clear perspective.
4. **Socialization and Community**: Some parents feel that a key part of education is developing social skills, which makes co-ops, public school, or group daycare appealing. Others might prioritize individual learning and home-based education. Thinking about how much interaction with peers you'd like your child to have can guide your decision.

5. **Financial Considerations**: Private schools, Montessori, and some daycare options can be costly, while public school is tuition-free. Calculate the potential costs and weigh them against what each option offers to determine the best value for your family.

Making Choices Free from External Pressure

It's natural to feel pressure from societal norms, friends, or family when making decisions about education. Each child and family is unique, and what works for one may not work for another. By focusing on your child's needs, family values, and lifestyle, you can make a confident choice that feels right for everyone.

It's important to give yourself grace. There is no perfect answer, and educational choices can evolve over time. If you choose one path and find it isn't working, most options allow for flexibility and adaptation as your child's needs change.

Whether you're drawn to homeschool, daycare, public or private school, the most important factor is choosing an environment where your child feels safe, supported, and encouraged to grow. Trust your instincts and remember that every family's journey is different.

Age-Appropriate Activities for Connecting with Kids

These activities focus on fostering developmental milestones while building meaningful connections with your child. From sensory play to nature exploration, these ideas emphasize organic, hands-on experiences that support growth and learning at every stage.

Infants (0-12 Months)

- **Skin-to-Skin and Gentle Massage**: These practices enhance bonding and promote relaxation. Infant massage can aid digestion, improve sleep, and support body awareness.
- **Sensory Play with Natural Materials**: Use items like soft fabrics, smooth wooden toys, and textured leaves to engage their senses. This supports tactile exploration, sensory processing, and motor skill development.
- **Nature Walks in a Carrier**: Being outdoors exposes babies to fresh air and natural sounds. Talking softly as you walk helps babies begin recognizing sounds and rhythm, supporting early language development.

Toddlers (1-3 Years)

- **Water and Sand Play**: Set up a small area for supervised water or sand play with cups and scoops. This fosters fine motor skills, sensory exploration, and problem-solving as they experiment with pouring and scooping.
- **Gardening Together**: Allow toddlers to plant seeds, water plants, or dig in the soil. Gardening builds fine motor skills and teaches basic cause-and-effect relationships while connecting them to nature.
- **Storytime and Picture Books**: Choose books with natural themes or realistic images. Reading together strengthens language skills and imagination while deepening your bond through close, cozy time.

Preschoolers (3-5 Years)

- **Nature Scavenger Hunts**: Create a list of natural items for them to find, like rocks, leaves, or pine cones. Scavenger hunts develop observation skills, curiosity, and an appreciation for the environment.
- **Baking Together**: Involve them in simple tasks like stirring, pouring, or rolling dough. Baking introduces basic math, fine motor skills, and patience while allowing time for fun conversations.
- **Yoga and Simple Mindfulness**: Introduce child-friendly yoga poses like "cat-cow" or "downward dog." Practicing yoga helps with physical coordination, focus, and emotional regulation, especially if combined with simple mindfulness exercises.

School-Age Children (6-10 Years)

- **Crafting with Natural Materials**: Encourage crafts using items like stones, leaves, and twigs to create artwork. These projects stimulate creativity, encourage recycling, and develop fine motor skills.
- **Nature Journals**: Go on nature walks, and have them draw or write about what they observe. Nature journaling supports observational skills, literacy, and self-expression while helping them connect deeply with their environment.
- **Cooking and Nutrition Education**: Teach them how to make simple, healthy snacks. Learning to prepare food fosters responsibility, healthy eating habits, and the basics of nutrition.

Tweens (10-12 Years)

- **DIY Projects with Eco-Friendly Materials**: Teach simple projects like making beeswax wraps, soap, or bath bombs. These hands-on activities are not only fun but also foster a sustainable mindset and practical skills.
- **Camping or Backyard Sleepovers**: Camping, even in the backyard, allows for star-gazing, storytelling, and independence. It encourages resilience, appreciation for nature, and bonding time with family.
- **Mindfulness and Emotional Check-Ins**: Engage in age-appropriate mindfulness practices and create space for talking about their emotions. Teaching self-regulation and open communication skills helps tweens navigate the transition into adolescence.

Teens (13+ Years)

- **Hiking or Adventure Days**: Plan day trips that involve exploration, like hiking or canoeing. These activities foster independence, build endurance, and provide time for meaningful conversations without distractions.
- **Cooking or Baking Complex Recipes**: Work on more advanced recipes together, such as sourdough bread or fermentation projects. This reinforces patience, skill-building, and provides a deeper understanding of nutrition and the joy of shared meals.
- **Volunteer Together**: Engage in community-based activities, like volunteering at a local farm or community garden. Volunteering instills values of empathy, connection, and responsibility while spending quality time together.

Fostering Connection Through Milestones and Natural Play

Each of these activities is designed to encourage natural development, align with developmental milestones, and strengthen the bond between parent and child. By embracing nature, creativity, and practical skills, you foster a sense of balance, independence, and a deep-rooted appreciation for the world.

Supporting Children Who Aren't Meeting Developmental Milestones: A Holistic Approach

If your child isn't reaching certain developmental milestones on time, it can be concerning. However, every child is unique, and delays don't always indicate a lasting issue. Here are supportive, natural steps crunchy moms can take to encourage healthy development while respecting their child's individual growth journey.

1. Observe and Listen Without Rushing to Conclusions

- **Take Note of Patterns**: If a milestone delay is observed, such as speech, motor skills, or social interactions, document when and how it appears. This helps track gradual progress and identify any recurring issues.
- **Remember the Variation**: Developmental milestones are general guidelines, not strict timelines. Every child grows at their own pace, and slight variations are normal. Focus on the overall pattern rather than individual benchmarks.

2. Nurture a Rich, Stimulating Environment

- **Engage in Sensory Play**: Sensory activities can promote motor skills, sensory processing, and even language development. Use items like water, sand, and natural objects to create a rich, tactile environment.

- **Encourage Open-Ended Play**: Unstructured play fosters problem-solving, creativity, and coordination. Natural toys like wooden blocks or art supplies give kids the freedom to explore, helping them build various developmental skills.
- **Nature Exposure**: Time outdoors is beneficial for physical development, sensory processing, and emotional regulation. Whether it's a walk in the park or gardening, nature play supports holistic growth.

3. Consider Nutrition and Gut Health

- **Nutrient-Rich Diet**: Ensure your child's diet is balanced, with whole foods rich in vitamins and minerals. Nutrients like omega-3s, B vitamins, iron, and protein are critical for brain and body development.
- **Probiotics and Gut Health**: A healthy gut influences cognitive and emotional development. Probiotics can support gut health, particularly if your child was born via C-section or has experienced digestive issues.
- **Limit Processed Foods and Sugars**: Processed foods, artificial colors, and refined sugars may contribute to behavioral and attention issues. Focusing on whole, nutrient-dense foods can make a significant difference.

4. Seek Natural Therapies

- **Speech and Occupational Therapy**: Holistic or integrative speech and occupational therapists can provide gentle, child-centered support. Therapies focused on play and sensory engagement respect your child's natural pace while building critical skills.

- **Physical Therapy for Movement and Coordination**: If there are gross motor delays, consider a physical therapist who takes a gentle approach, incorporating nature and play-based exercises.
- **Consider Complementary Modalities**: Gentle techniques like craniosacral therapy, music therapy, or animal-assisted therapy can support development, especially for children sensitive to conventional therapies.

5. Practice Patience and Gentle Encouragement

- **Foster a Low-Pressure Environment**: Create a nurturing atmosphere where your child feels encouraged without feeling pressure. Avoid comparing them to siblings or peers, and celebrate small achievements, building their confidence.
- **Model Skills through Play**: Engage in activities that allow your child to observe and imitate. For example, if speech is delayed, narrate your daily routines and include them in conversations. Modeling helps kids absorb language and behavior through positive examples.

6. Use Natural Resources for Emotional Support

- **Focus on Emotional Wellness**: Developmental delays can impact children's self-esteem, so use calming practices like mindfulness, breathing exercises, and guided meditation. These help kids build emotional resilience.

- **Flower Essences for Support**: Consider Bach Flower Remedies like Mimulus (for fearfulness) or Larch (for confidence) to support children who may feel frustrated or discouraged by developmental challenges.

7. Know When to Seek Support

- **Trust Your Intuition**: If you have concerns about a specific area of development, consider consulting with a pediatrician or developmental specialist. Look for practitioners who respect holistic values and will approach the situation with a whole-child perspective.
- **Explore Community Resources**: Connect with local or online support groups for other parents, particularly those that share a natural or holistic approach. Shared experiences can provide comfort and practical advice, reminding you that you're not alone.

Embracing Your Child's Unique Path

If your child isn't meeting milestones on time, remember that they are on their own unique journey. Holistic, supportive approaches can gently encourage growth, offering positive support without imposing external expectations. By nurturing their physical, emotional, and cognitive development with patience and love, you're providing them with a strong foundation for future growth and confidence.

Anecdotes of Children Discovering Their Talents through Play

One mother shared the story of her son, Leo, who spent hours every afternoon building intricate cities with blocks and Lego pieces. There was no formal instruction—just pure, unstructured play. Over time, his parents realized that Leo's passion for building had transformed into a keen interest in architecture. His natural curiosity, given the space to flourish, revealed a potential future career path that they might have otherwise overlooked.

Another family shared how their daughter, Sophie, discovered a love for art during her free time at home. Initially, Sophie's parents had enrolled her in various extracurricular activities, including soccer and dance, but they noticed that she seemed happiest when she was simply drawing or painting at the kitchen table. Eventually, they encouraged her to spend more time exploring art, and her creativity blossomed.

Families Finding Balance between Structure and Free Growth

The Davis family had always been dedicated to ensuring their children had a well-rounded education, enrolling them in after-school programs for sports, music, and tutoring. However, they began to notice that their children seemed exhausted and lacked enthusiasm for many of these activities. After some reflection, they decided to scale back on structured activities and give their kids more free time for creative play. The change was remarkable. Their children became more engaged in their schoolwork, were happier at home, and found joy in activities they chose for themselves. The balance they struck between structure and freedom allowed their children's natural growth to flourish.

Nurturing natural growth honors your child's unique journey. By giving them the space to explore, play, and develop at their own pace, you're fostering resilience, creativity, and a sense of well-being that will serve them for life. Trust in the process and allow your child to grow into the best version of themselves, free from unnecessary pressure or intervention.

By supporting your child's natural growth, you allow them to reach their full potential in a holistic, well-balanced way. Rather than rushing or forcing development, you provide the nurturing environment they need to thrive on their own terms.

Next, we explore the importance of community and support systems in raising well-balanced children. In the following chapter, we'll take a closer look at how building a strong support network, from family to friends, plays a vital role in a child's growth and development. After all, it truly takes a village.

9

Building a Supportive Community

The old adage "it takes a village" has never been more relevant than in today's fast-paced, often disconnected world. Raising children is no easy task, and having a strong community of like-minded individuals to lean on can make all the difference. In modern society, building a support system is essential, not just for emotional and practical help but for sharing wisdom and reinforcing holistic parenting practices. Whether it's advice on natural remedies, emotional encouragement during tough times, or simply the feeling of belonging, a supportive community is a vital resource for both parents and children.

A strong community plays a crucial role in raising healthy, well-balanced children, aligning with the principles of holistic parenting. Through shared experiences, collective wisdom, and mutual support, parents and children alike benefit from being part of a community that values natural health, non-toxic living, and conscious parenting.

The Benefits of a Community Network

Emotional and Practical Support

Navigating the world of holistic parenting can sometimes

feel overwhelming, especially when mainstream options or advice don't align with your values. A like-minded community can offer the emotional and practical support you need on this journey. Whether you're struggling with a parenting challenge, seeking natural health solutions, or simply need reassurance, a community provides a safe space to share your concerns and gain perspective.

For many parents, having access to practical advice from others who share similar values can be invaluable. Whether it's learning about the best non-toxic products for your home, understanding the nuances of alternative health practices, or finding support during tough times, a community helps ease the burden of decision-making. It provides emotional encouragement when the journey feels isolating, offering a sense of belonging that is often missing in today's individualistic culture.

Sharing Knowledge and Resources

One of the greatest strengths of a community is the collective wisdom it offers. Parents who are further along in their holistic health journey can share their experiences, offering guidance and recommendations to those just starting out. This exchange of knowledge is especially powerful in areas like alternative health practices, non-toxic living, and natural remedies, where mainstream advice may be limited.

In addition, being part of a community opens up resources that might otherwise be difficult to access. Whether it's sharing bulk orders of organic produce, participating in natural remedy workshops, or swapping knowledge about local practitioners who specialize in holistic care, a community amplifies your ability to make informed, conscious choices for your family.

Finding and Building Your Community

Where to Start

Finding or building your own supportive community may feel daunting, but there are plenty of opportunities to connect with others who share your values. Here are a few ways to get started:

- **Local Meetups:** Look for local parenting groups focused on holistic health, organic living, or natural remedies. Many cities have community centers or co-ops that host events and gatherings for families with similar values.
- **Online Forums and Social Media Groups:** In the digital age, it's easier than ever to find online communities. Search for Facebook groups, forums, or websites dedicated to holistic parenting, natural remedies, or non-toxic living. These virtual spaces can provide a wealth of information and support, and they often lead to real-world connections.
- **Alternative Health Networks:** Many cities have holistic health practitioners or natural living groups that host workshops or seminars. These events are great places to meet like-minded parents and learn more about integrating natural practices into your lifestyle.

If you can't find a community that fits your needs, consider starting your own. Creating a local organic food co-op, hosting playdates with a natural health focus, or organizing wellness workshops for parents can be great ways to bring like-minded families together.

Nurturing a Sense of Community in Children

It's not just parents who benefit from a strong community—children also thrive when they feel connected to others. Growing up in a supportive, collaborative environment teaches children important social skills, like empathy, cooperation, and communication. When children see their parents actively participating in a community, they learn the value of relationships and understand that they are part of something larger than themselves.

Involvement in community activities—whether it's participating in a local gardening project, attending family wellness workshops, or simply playing with other children who share similar values—helps children develop a sense of belonging. It also fosters collaboration and teamwork, essential skills for emotional and social development.

Creating Your Own Community: Building Support from the Ground Up

For parents embracing holistic and natural parenting practices, finding like-minded individuals can be invaluable. However, in some areas, established communities focused on natural health and holistic parenting may be scarce. If you find yourself without a local network, building your own supportive community is not only possible but can be incredibly rewarding.

1. **Start Small and Set Clear Intentions**

- **Define Your Purpose**: Consider what kind of support you want from your community—whether it's shared learning, playdates focused on natural practices, or collaborative workshops on holistic health.
- **Choose a Platform to Connect**: Begin by creating a private group on social media platforms, such as Facebook or Instagram, where you can invite others to join and engage in discussions, share resources, and plan meetups.

2. **Reach Out to Potential Members**

- **Advertise Your Group**: Share flyers in local health food stores, holistic wellness centers, and libraries. You can also post on local community boards or websites like Nextdoor.
- **Leverage Existing Networks**: Reach out to other parents you know from playgroups, school, or community events. Let them know you're starting a group that embraces natural parenting practices, and encourage them to invite friends who may be interested.

3. Host Initial Meetups

- **Plan an Introductory Gathering**: Host a small, informal get-together at a park, community center, or your home. This can include activities like a nature walk, potluck with whole foods, or a discussion on topics like non-toxic household products or DIY herbal remedies.
- **Use Virtual Meetups**: If in-person gatherings aren't feasible, arrange virtual meetups using platforms like Zoom. Online sessions can include group discussions, workshops, or guest speakers on holistic topics.

4. Create Shared Activities and Themes

- **Educational Workshops**: Organize events focused on shared learning, such as workshops on making homemade herbal tinctures, meditation for kids, or baby-led weaning.
- **Playdates with Purpose**: Plan playdates that integrate natural activities like gardening, making crafts with natural materials, or exploring nature trails.
- **Seasonal Celebrations**: Celebrate seasonal changes with activities like solstice gatherings, autumn harvest parties,

or spring planting events. These traditions foster a sense of rhythm and community among families.

5. Maintain Engagement and Growth

- **Regular Communication**: Keep members engaged by posting regularly, sharing helpful resources, and asking for input on upcoming events. Consistent communication fosters a sense of belonging.
- **Encourage Participation**: Rotate leadership roles for organizing meetups or leading workshops. This involvement helps create a shared sense of ownership and commitment to the group.
- **Be Inclusive but True to Your Values**: Welcome diverse members while staying aligned with the core principles of natural, holistic parenting. This balance helps maintain a supportive and focused environment.

6. Expand with Purpose

- **Collaborate with Local Businesses**: Partner with health food stores, wellness practitioners, and yoga studios to co-host events or offer group discounts. This not only enriches your community but also draws attention to holistic health practices.
- **Create a Resource Library**: Compile a shared list of books, articles, and recommended practitioners that align with holistic and natural practices, available to all members.
- **Host Guest Speakers**: Invite local or virtual experts in natural health, child development, or sustainable living to share their knowledge with the group.

The Challenges of Being Crunchy: Navigating Unsupportive Friends and Family

Choosing a holistic and natural parenting path, or being a "crunchy" parent, often means stepping outside of conventional norms. This decision, while fulfilling and aligned with your values, can come with significant challenges. One of the most difficult aspects is facing criticism from friends, family, or even partners who may not understand or support your choices.

Understanding the Weight of Others' Opinions

When friends and family don't share your views on natural health practices, the result can be feelings of isolation, frustration, and self-doubt. It's especially tough when the people you care about question your decisions or label your practices as extreme or unfounded. Experiences like being called a "homeopathic cultist" or dealing with confrontational behavior from loved ones can make it feel as though you're constantly defending your beliefs.

Advice for Conquering Criticism

1. **Stay Grounded in Your Beliefs**

- **Educate Yourself**: The more informed you are about your choices, the more confident you will be in defending them when needed. Continue learning from trusted sources, holistic health leaders, and other parents on the same path.
- **Reflect on Your "Why"**: Remind yourself of why you chose this path—whether it's because of personal health experiences, your children's well-being, or the values you hold. This will help you stay strong when faced with criticism.

1. **Set Boundaries**

- **Communicate Your Limits**: Let friends and family know that while you respect their views, you expect the same in return. Explain that debates or confrontations about your lifestyle choices are not welcome if they don't come from a place of understanding.
- **Protect Your Peace**: If someone repeatedly undermines or belittles your parenting, consider taking a step back from that relationship or limiting discussions on topics you know will lead to conflict.

1. **Find Your Support System**

- **Join or Build a Community**: Surrounding yourself with like-minded people can be empowering. When you don't have this community locally, building your own network (such as the Holistic Leaders Collective) can provide you with the support and encouragement you need. Sharing experiences, advice, and victories with those who understand your choices reinforces your confidence.
- **Lean on Trusted Allies**: Seek out friends or family members who, even if they don't share your beliefs, are willing to listen and be supportive. Having someone in your corner can make a huge difference when facing skepticism from others.

1. **Respond with Grace and Confidence**

- **Choose When to Engage**: You don't always need to defend or explain your choices. Sometimes, a simple, "This is what works for us," is enough to set the boundary. Not every criticism needs a response.

- **Respond Calmly**: If you choose to explain, do so with composure. Present your decisions as thoughtful choices based on research, experience, and what you believe is best for your family.

1. **Accept That Not Everyone Will Understand**

- **Release the Need for Approval**: Recognize that not everyone will be open to your choices, and that's okay. Your role isn't to convince everyone—it's to do what's right for you and your family.
- **Embrace Your Journey**: Acknowledge that being a pioneer in your circle means facing resistance. Remember, your journey may inspire others in ways you won't immediately see, and your steadfastness could plant seeds of curiosity and change.

Turning Challenges into Motivation

Your experiences, even the challenging ones, can lead to growth and purpose. For instance, enduring harsh criticism from a partner about your holistic choices may be painful but can also ignite a drive to create spaces where others can find support. This is what led to the creation of the **Holistic Leaders Collective**, a community that champions understanding, learning, and empowerment.

Embracing the crunchy lifestyle means choosing to walk a path that may not be widely understood or accepted—but it's one that is true to your beliefs and your family's well being. Stand tall, find your people, and let your journey be both your shield and your inspiration.

The Power of Community You Create

Creating your own community may seem daunting at first, but it's a powerful way to connect with like-minded parents and build a supportive network centered on holistic living. The relationships and shared experiences that come from these efforts provide not only practical benefits but also emotional support as you navigate the journey of natural parenting together.

The Story of a Group of Mothers Who Created a Local Organic Food Co-op

In a small town in Oregon, a group of mothers, frustrated by the limited access to affordable organic produce, decided to take matters into their own hands. They formed a local organic food co-op, pooling their resources to buy in bulk directly from farmers. What started as a small group of families sharing weekly produce orders soon grew into a thriving community network. Not only did they create access to fresh, organic food, but they also hosted workshops on canning, gardening, and meal prepping. The co-op became more than just a source of food—it became a support system, a place where mothers could share tips, offer encouragement, and bond over their shared commitment to healthy living.

A Humorous Account of the Power of Shared Parenting Experiences

Sometimes, the power of community shines through in the small moments. One mother shared a funny story about how, during a particularly challenging week of sleepless nights with her newborn, she posted a question in her local holistic parenting group asking for advice on natural sleep aids. She was inundated with suggestions, but one piece of advice stood out: "Try swaddling the baby while listening to white noise... or, if that doesn't work, just accept that you'll never sleep again!" The humor and honesty in that response made her laugh out loud, and it reminded her that she wasn't alone in the struggles of parenting. Sometimes, knowing that other parents are going through the same challenges is all the comfort you need.

The power of community is transformative. Being part of a supportive network offers parents emotional reassurance, practical advice, and shared experiences that reinforce the values of holistic parenting. Whether it's through in-person meetups or online forums, connecting with a like-minded community amplifies your ability to raise healthy, well-balanced children.

Community support is a critical pillar in the holistic health journey. It provides the encouragement and accountability needed to stay on track and to make the best decisions for your family's health and well-being. In the end, we are stronger together, and the shared wisdom of a community can make all the difference.

Next, we'll explore the practical side of using natural remedies for common childhood ailments. In the following chapter, we'll dive into how natural solutions can be used safely and effectively to manage everyday health issues.

10

Natural Remedies for Everyday Ailments

Imagine opening your medicine cabinet and instead of rows of over-the-counter medications, you see shelves lined with herbal tinctures, essential oils, homeopathic remedies, and natural solutions that have been trusted for generations. In a world where conventional medicine often dominates, it can be empowering to turn to nature to care for everyday childhood ailments. Natural remedies offer a holistic approach to managing common health issues, from colds and fevers to digestive discomfort, empowering parents to provide safe, gentle relief for their children.

Everyday childhood ailments, such as colds, fevers, stomach aches, and minor injuries, can often be effectively managed with natural remedies. By understanding how to use herbs, essential oils, homeopathy, and other natural solutions, parents can take control of their child's health in a holistic and empowering way. This chapter explores common natural remedies and when to balance them with conventional medicine.

Common Natural Remedies

Herbal Alternatives to OTC Medications

Herbs have been used for centuries to treat a wide range of common health issues, and many parents are rediscovering their healing power as a natural alternative to over-the-counter (OTC) medications. Here are a few herbal remedies that can be helpful for everyday ailments:

Chamomile: Chamomile is renowned for its calming properties and can be used to soothe an upset stomach, relieve teething pain, or help children relax before bedtime. A cup of chamomile tea or a few drops of chamomile tincture can ease tension and support restful sleep.

Elderberry: Rich in antioxidants and vitamins, elderberry syrup is a go-to remedy for boosting the immune system and treating colds and flu. Studies have shown that elderberry can help reduce the duration and severity of cold symptoms when taken at the first sign of illness.

Ginger: Ginger is excellent for digestive discomfort and nausea. Whether your child is dealing with motion sickness or a stomach bug, ginger tea or a small amount of ginger syrup can settle the stomach and relieve nausea effectively.

Echinacea: This immune-boosting herb is commonly used to help prevent or shorten the duration of colds and respiratory infections. Echinacea can be taken as a tea or in tincture form to provide added support during flu season.

Peppermint: Peppermint is a powerful herb for soothing digestive issues and relieving headaches. A warm cup of peppermint tea can alleviate bloating and stomach cramps, while diluted peppermint oil can be applied to the temples for tension headaches.

Slippery Elm: Slippery elm has a soothing effect on the digestive tract and can help relieve symptoms of indigestion or acid reflux. It is also effective for sore throats and can be consumed as a lozenge or mixed with water to form a soothing drink.

Lavender: Lavender is well-known for its relaxing aroma and is often used to promote restful sleep and reduce anxiety. A few drops of lavender essential oil in a diffuser or a warm bath can create a calming environment for children.

Calendula: This herb is excellent for soothing skin irritations, cuts, and rashes. Calendula can be applied topically as a cream or ointment to promote healing and reduce inflammation.

Marshmallow Root: Known for its mucilaginous properties, marshmallow root can help soothe an irritated gut lining and alleviate constipation. It can also be used to calm sore throats when prepared as a tea or tincture.

Thyme: Thyme is effective for respiratory health and can help reduce coughing and congestion. Thyme tea or a diluted thyme oil steam inhalation can provide relief during colds and coughs.

Valerian Root: Valerian root is used to aid sleep and reduce anxiety. A small dose in tea or tincture form can help calm a restless child and promote a peaceful night's sleep.

Lemon Balm: Lemon balm is a gentle herb that helps soothe nervousness and reduce hyperactivity. It can be made into tea or added as a tincture to help children feel calm and focused.

Licorice Root: This herb is beneficial for soothing sore throats and boosting immune function. It can be prepared as a tea or taken as a syrup for children over the age of two.

Fennel: Fennel is excellent for easing gas, bloating, and digestive discomfort. Fennel tea can be given to children to support digestion after meals.

Horehound: Horehound is used for treating coughs and sore throats due to its natural expectorant properties. A homemade horehound syrup can help soothe an irritated throat and clear mucus.

Nettle: Nettle is a nutrient-rich herb that helps with seasonal allergies and provides a boost in vitamins and minerals. Nettle tea or tincture can be given to support immune function and reduce allergy symptoms.

Dandelion: Dandelion supports healthy digestion and liver function. Dandelion tea can be mildly detoxifying and beneficial for children's digestive health.

Turmeric: Turmeric is renowned for its anti-inflammatory properties and can be used for joint pain or inflammation. A small amount of turmeric mixed with honey or added to smoothies can offer gentle support.

Rosemary: Rosemary can help improve concentration and boost memory. Diffusing rosemary essential oil or adding it to meals can support cognitive function and promote alertness.

Oregano: Oregano is known for its powerful antibacterial and antiviral properties. A diluted oregano oil or oregano tea can help fight infections and boost immune support.

Cinnamon: Cinnamon has natural antibacterial properties and can help regulate blood sugar levels. A sprinkle of cinnamon on oatmeal or warm milk can support digestion and immune health.

Garlic: Garlic is a natural immune booster with antiviral and antibacterial properties. It can be added to meals or taken in a milder form, such as garlic oil, for children to help prevent colds.

Hibiscus: High in vitamin C, hibiscus tea can help boost the immune system and lower blood pressure. It's a tasty, tangy drink that kids often enjoy cold.

Ginseng: Ginseng supports energy levels and cognitive function. A mild ginseng tea can be offered in small doses for older children to support mental clarity.

Yarrow: Yarrow is used to reduce fever and aid in wound healing. A warm yarrow tea can help manage fevers naturally.

These herbal remedies provide gentle, effective support for your child's body without the side effects that often accompany synthetic medications. Always consult a qualified herbalist or healthcare provider to ensure the appropriate usage and dosage for children.

Safe Use of Essential Oils and Tinctures

Essential oils and herbal tinctures are potent natural remedies, but they must be used safely, especially with children. Here are some best practices for using these remedies:

- **Essential Oils**: Always dilute essential oils before applying them to your child's skin. A safe dilution ratio is typically 1-2 drops of essential oil per teaspoon of a carrier oil, such as coconut or almond oil. Oils like lavender, tea tree, and eucalyptus are popular for treating issues like colds, skin irritations, and sleep disturbances, but some oils should be avoided with young children (like peppermint for babies under two years old).
- **Herbal Tinctures**: Tinctures are concentrated liquid extracts of herbs, typically preserved in alcohol or glycerin. Glycerin-based tinctures are generally safer for children. Always consult with a qualified herbalist or follow the dosage recommendations on the tincture bottle to ensure safe use.

These remedies can be powerful allies in maintaining your child's health, but always practice caution and use the correct dilutions and dosages to avoid any adverse effects.

25 Commonly Used Essential Oils for Kids: Uses, Safety, and Directions

1. Lavender

- **Uses**: Calms anxiety, promotes sleep, and soothes skin irritations.
- **Safety**: Safe for children 6 months+.
- **Directions**: Diffuse or dilute 1-2 drops in carrier oil and apply to skin.
- **Carrier Oil**: Coconut oil, jojoba oil.

2. Roman Chamomile

- **Uses**: Eases colic, soothes teething pain, reduces stress, and aids sleep.
- **Safety**: Safe for children 6 months+.
- **Directions**: Diffuse or dilute in carrier oil for gentle massage.
- **Carrier Oil**: Almond oil, olive oil.

3. Frankincense

- **Uses**: Supports immune function, promotes wound healing, and calms the mind.
- **Safety**: Safe for children 2+ years.
- **Directions**: Dilute 1 drop in carrier oil and apply to the chest or feet.
- **Carrier Oil**: Coconut oil, avocado oil.

4. Tea Tree (Melaleuca)

- **Uses**: Antibacterial, anti fungal, helps with skin irritations.
- **Safety**: Safe for children 2+ years (avoid using near the face).
- **Directions**: Dilute in carrier oil and apply to affected areas.
- **Carrier Oil**: Jojoba oil, grapeseed oil.

5. Sweet Orange

- **Uses**: Uplifts mood, reduces anxiety, aids digestion.
- **Safety**: Safe for children 6 months+ (avoid sun exposure after use due to phototoxicity).
- **Directions**: Diffuse or dilute for massage.
- **Carrier Oil**: Coconut oil, almond oil.

6. Lemon

- **Uses**: Cleanses air, boosts immunity, improves mood.
- **Safety**: Safe for children 6 months+ (phototoxic, avoid sun exposure).
- **Directions**: Diffuse or dilute for topical use.
- **Carrier Oil**: Olive oil, grapeseed oil.

7. Eucalyptus Radiata

- **Uses**: Clears congestion, supports respiratory health.
- **Safety**: Safe for children 2+ years (use with caution in younger children).
- **Directions**: Dilute and apply to chest or diffuse.
- **Carrier Oil**: Coconut oil, olive oil.

8. Peppermint

- **Uses**: Relieves headaches, clears nasal congestion, soothes upset stomach.
- **Safety**: Safe for children 6+ years (avoid face and chest of younger children).
- **Directions**: Dilute and apply to the temples or feet.
- **Carrier Oil**: Almond oil, olive oil.

9. Cedarwood

- **Uses**: Calms anxiety, promotes sleep, repels insects.
- **Safety**: Safe for children 6 months+.
- **Directions**: Diffuse or dilute and apply to skin.
- **Carrier Oil**: Coconut oil, jojoba oil.

10. Geranium

- **Uses**: Balances mood, promotes skin healing.
- **Safety**: Safe for children 2+ years.
- **Directions**: Dilute and apply to skin for dry patches or rashes.
- **Carrier Oil**: Almond oil, grapeseed oil.

11. Helichrysum

- **Uses**: Heals wounds, reduces inflammation, soothes skin irritations.
- **Safety**: Safe for children 2+ years.
- **Directions**: Dilute and apply to wounds or skin irritations.
- **Carrier Oil**: Olive oil, avocado oil.

12. Ylang Ylang

- **Uses**: Calms anxiety, promotes relaxation, balances mood.
- **Safety**: Safe for children 2+ years.
- **Directions**: Diffuse or dilute for topical use.
- **Carrier Oil**: Jojoba oil, coconut oil.

13. Sandalwood

- **Uses**: Calms the mind, reduces anxiety, supports skin health.
- **Safety**: Safe for children 2+ years.
- **Directions**: Diffuse or dilute for massage.
- **Carrier Oil**: Almond oil, olive oil.

14. Clary Sage

- **Uses**: Relieves stress, balances hormones, and calms nerves.
- **Safety**: Safe for children 2+ years.
- **Directions**: Dilute and apply to skin or diffuse.
- **Carrier Oil**: Coconut oil, grapeseed oil.

15. Roman Chamomile

- **Uses**: Soothes teething pain, reduces anxiety, and improves sleep.
- **Safety**: Safe for children 6 months+.
- **Directions**: Diffuse or dilute and apply to skin.
- **Carrier Oil**: Almond oil, jojoba oil.

16. Patchouli

- **Uses**: Promotes skin healing, reduces inflammation, balances mood.

- **Safety**: Safe for children 2+ years.
- **Directions**: Diffuse or dilute for topical use.
- **Carrier Oil**: Olive oil, jojoba oil.

17. Marjoram

- **Uses**: Relieves muscle pain, promotes relaxation, soothes digestive issues.
- **Safety**: Safe for children 6 months+.
- **Directions**: Dilute and massage into muscles or abdomen.
- **Carrier Oil**: Coconut oil, almond oil.

18. Vetiver

- **Uses**: Calms the mind, promotes restful sleep, soothes anxiety.
- **Safety**: Safe for children 2+ years.
- **Directions**: Diffuse or dilute for application.
- **Carrier Oil**: Jojoba oil, avocado oil.

19. Melissa (Lemon Balm)

- **Uses**: Eases anxiety, promotes relaxation, supports the immune system.
- **Safety**: Safe for children 2+ years.
- **Directions**: Diffuse or dilute for massage.
- **Carrier Oil**: Coconut oil, grapeseed oil.

20. Copaiba

- **Uses**: Reduces inflammation, supports emotional balance.
- **Safety**: Safe for children 2+ years.
- **Directions**: Dilute and apply to skin or diffuse.
- **Carrier Oil**: Almond oil, olive oil.

21. Bergamot

- **Uses**: Uplifts mood, reduces stress, supports digestion.
- **Safety**: Safe for children 2+ years (avoid sun exposure due to phototoxicity).
- **Directions**: Diffuse or dilute for topical use.
- **Carrier Oil**: Almond oil, grapeseed oil.

22. Spearmint

- **Uses**: Eases nausea, promotes focus, relieves digestive issues.
- **Safety**: Safe for children 2+ years.
- **Directions**: Diffuse or dilute for topical use.
- **Carrier Oil**: Jojoba oil, coconut oil.

23. Thyme

- **Uses**: Antibacterial, supports immune and respiratory health.
- **Safety**: Safe for children 6+ years (dilute well for topical use).
- **Directions**: Diffuse or apply diluted to chest.
- **Carrier Oil**: Olive oil, grapeseed oil.

24. Lemon Balm (Melissa)

- **Uses**: Reduces anxiety, promotes sleep, supports immunity.
- **Safety**: Safe for children 2+ years.
- **Directions**: Diffuse or apply diluted to skin.
- **Carrier Oil**: Coconut oil, jojoba oil.

25. Fennel (Sweet)

- **Uses**: Supports digestion, reduces gas and bloating.
- **Safety**: Safe for children 2+ years (use sparingly).
- **Directions**: Dilute and apply to the abdomen or diffuse.
- **Carrier Oil**: Olive oil, almond oil.

Safety Considerations

- **Dilution Ratios for Kids**:
- For infants (6+ months): 1 drop of essential oil per 1 tablespoon of carrier oil.
- For toddlers (1-2 years): 1-2 drops per tablespoon of carrier oil.
- For children 2-6 years: 1 drop per teaspoon of carrier oil.
- **Common Carrier Oils**:
- **Coconut oil**: Moisturizing and absorbs well.
- **Jojoba oil**: Non-greasy and hypoallergenic.
- **Almond oil**: Nourishes the skin and is gentle for children.
- **Olive oil**: Great for moisturizing and soothing.

Common Carrier Oils and Their Benefits

1. **Coconut Oil**: Known for its antibacterial and anti fungal properties, coconut oil is highly moisturizing and excellent for soothing dry or irritated skin.

2. **Sweet Almond Oil**: Rich in vitamins A, E, and fatty acids, this light oil is great for sensitive skin and helps with moisturizing and reducing skin inflammation.
3. **Jojoba Oil**: Closely resembles the skin's natural sebum, making it suitable for all skin types. It absorbs easily and helps balance oil production.
4. **Grapeseed Oil**: A lightweight oil that is non-greasy and rich in antioxidants. Ideal for oily skin, it helps tone and tighten the skin.
5. **Olive Oil**: High in antioxidants and vitamins, olive oil is beneficial for deep moisturizing and soothing dry or damaged skin.
6. **Avocado Oil**: Packed with vitamins A, D, and E, it's highly nourishing and helps support skin elasticity and repair.
7. **Sunflower Oil**: A light oil rich in vitamin E, it's perfect for sensitive skin and provides a protective barrier to lock in moisture.
8. **Argan Oil**: Known as "liquid gold," argan oil is rich in vitamin E and fatty acids. It helps nourish and soften the skin and hair.
9. **Rosehip Seed Oil**: High in vitamins A and C, this oil is known for its ability to reduce scars, fine lines, and pigmentation.
10. **Apricot Kernel Oil**: A gentle oil that is rich in vitamins A and E, making it great for sensitive or mature skin.
11. **Sesame Oil**: Contains natural anti-inflammatory properties and antioxidants that help with skin regeneration.
12. **Castor Oil**: Known for its deep moisturizing properties and antibacterial qualities. It is often used in hair care and for treating minor skin irritations.
13. **Hemp Seed Oil**: Contains omega-3 and omega-6 fatty

acids, providing anti-inflammatory benefits and supporting skin hydration.

14. **Macadamia Nut Oil**: Rich in oleic and palmitoleic acids, it helps restore and soften dry or mature skin.
15. **Tamanu Oil**: Famous for its wound-healing and anti-inflammatory properties, tamanu oil is used for scar reduction and skin regeneration.

Essential Oil Safety and Allergic Reactions: Important Guidelines

What to Do if Your Child Has an Allergic Reaction to Essential Oils: Even when used carefully, essential oils can sometimes cause allergic reactions in children. Signs of an allergic reaction may include redness, itching, swelling, or rashes. If your child shows any of these symptoms:

- **Stop Use Immediately**: Cease using the oil and wash the affected area with mild soap and water.
- **Apply a Carrier Oil**: Dilute the area with a carrier oil, such as coconut or olive oil, to help reduce irritation.
- **Monitor for Severe Reactions**: If symptoms worsen or breathing difficulties occur, seek immediate medical attention.
- **Consult a Professional**: Reach out to a healthcare provider or holistic practitioner for guidance on future use.

Essential Oils to Avoid for Pregnant Women and Children: Some essential oils should be avoided due to their strong effects and potential risks. These include:

- **For Pregnant Women**: Avoid oils such as clary sage, rosemary, and wintergreen, as they may stimulate contractions or have other adverse effects.
- **For Children**: Essential oils like peppermint (for children under 6), eucalyptus (for children under 10), and tea tree oil should be used with caution or avoided altogether due to potential respiratory or skin sensitivities.

Using Essential Oils as Natural Cleaners

Essential oils can be used safely to create non-toxic household cleaners that are effective and smell great. Combine a few drops of lemon, lavender, or tea tree oil with water and white vinegar for an all-purpose cleaner. Always store homemade solutions out of reach of children.

By following these safety practices and knowing when to use or avoid certain oils, you can enjoy the benefits of essential oils while ensuring the well-being of your family.

Herbal Tinctures Every Mom Should Keep on Hand

Herbal tinctures are concentrated liquid extracts made from herbs, offering a convenient way to support your family's health naturally. They are easy to use, fast-acting, and effective for a variety of common ailments. Here's a list of essential tinctures that moms should consider having on hand:

1. **Elderberry Tincture**: This tincture is essential for immune support and helps fight off colds and flu. When taken at the first sign of symptoms, elderberry tincture can reduce the severity and duration of illnesses, making it a must-have

during cold and flu season.

2. **Chamomile Tincture**: Renowned for its calming properties, chamomile tincture is great for easing anxiety, promoting restful sleep, and soothing digestive issues. It's safe for kids and can also help relieve teething pain and upset stomachs.
3. **Echinacea Tincture**: Known for boosting the immune system, echinacea tincture can help prevent or shorten the duration of colds and other respiratory infections. It's an excellent go-to for added support during seasonal changes.
4. **Ginger Tincture**: Ginger is well-known for its ability to alleviate nausea, motion sickness, and digestive discomfort. A few drops of ginger tincture can settle an upset stomach and relieve mild indigestion, making it a staple for families on the go.
5. **Peppermint Tincture**: Perfect for digestive issues such as bloating, gas, and upset stomachs, peppermint tincture can also be applied topically (diluted) for headaches. It's refreshing and effective for easing tension.
6. **Lemon Balm Tincture**: Lemon balm is a gentle herb that helps reduce stress, promote relaxation, and calm hyperactivity. This tincture is ideal for children who experience restlessness or have trouble winding down before bedtime.
7. **Valerian Root Tincture**: Valerian root tincture is known for promoting deep, restful sleep and easing mild anxiety. Use sparingly and as needed, as it's strong and best for short-term support.
8. **Calendula Tincture**: Calendula tincture is excellent for treating minor cuts, scrapes, and skin irritations. With its antibacterial and anti-inflammatory properties, it can

be used topically or taken internally for overall skin health.

9. **Slippery Elm Tincture**: This soothing herb supports the digestive tract and helps with indigestion, acid reflux, and constipation. Slippery elm tincture is gentle enough for children, providing relief without harsh side effects.
10. **Ashwagandha Tincture**: Ashwagandha is an adaptogenic herb that supports stress management and adrenal health. It's particularly beneficial for moms looking to reduce stress and boost their energy naturally.
11. **Nettle Tincture**: Nettle tincture is rich in vitamins and minerals, making it great for overall health support. It also provides relief from seasonal allergies and helps strengthen the immune system.
12. **Turmeric Tincture**: Known for its powerful anti-inflammatory properties, turmeric tincture can help reduce joint pain and boost immune response. It's a versatile addition to any holistic medicine cabinet.
13. **Licorice Root Tincture**: This tincture is beneficial for soothing sore throats and supporting respiratory health. Licorice root also aids in boosting immunity and calming digestive discomfort.
14. **Hawthorn Tincture**: Hawthorn is supportive of cardiovascular health and can help ease mild anxiety. It's a gentle herb that promotes heart health and emotional well-being.
15. **Fennel Tincture**: Fennel tincture is excellent for relieving gas, bloating, and digestive discomfort, making it perfect for moms with infants experiencing colic or children who struggle with indigestion.

Why Tinctures Are Essential

Herbal tinctures provide gentle, effective support for various health needs without the side effects that often accompany synthetic medications. They can be taken alone or added to water or juice for easier consumption. Always consult with a qualified herbalist or healthcare provider to ensure proper usage and dosage for children.

Homeopathy: A Gentle and Holistic Approach

Homeopathy: A Gentle Approach to Childhood Ailments

Homeopathy is a system of medicine that uses highly diluted substances to stimulate the body's natural healing processes. It's based on the principle of "like cures like," meaning that a substance that causes symptoms in a healthy person can be used to treat similar symptoms in a sick person. Homeopathy is considered safe for children as the remedies are non-toxic, non-addictive, and have no known side effects.

Understanding Materia Medica and Repertory

Central to homeopathy are the Materia Medica and the Repertory, two essential tools used to determine the most appropriate remedy:

Materia Medica: This is a comprehensive reference that lists homeopathic remedies and describes their properties, including the symptoms they address. Each entry provides detailed information about how a remedy affects the body, mind, and emotions. For example, Arnica in the Materia Medica would include its use for trauma, swelling, and bruising.

Repertory: The Repertory is an index or database that helps match specific symptoms to potential remedies. It is organized by symptoms (e.g., fever, teething pain, irritability) and guides users to remedies listed in the Materia Medica. Parents and practitioners use the Repertory to pinpoint which remedy best fits the unique set of symptoms a child is experiencing.

Common Homeopathic Remedies for Kids

1. Arnica: Useful for bumps, bruises, and injuries; reduces swelling and speeds up healing.

2. Chamomilla: Ideal for teething pain, irritability, and restlessness.

3. Belladonna: Effective for sudden high fevers, inflammation, and headaches.

4. Pulsatilla: Helps with colds that produce thick, yellow mucus and comforts weepy children.

5. Aconite: Used for sudden onset of colds or fevers, especially after exposure to cold weather.

6. Calcarea Carbonica: Supports children who are slow to reach developmental milestones and for teething issues.

7. Nux Vomica: Assists with digestive upsets, nausea, and constipation.

8. Ferrum Phosphoricum: A gentle remedy for early stages of inflammation, mild fevers, and colds.

9. Silicea: Used for recurrent infections, such as earaches, and to support the immune system.

10. Gelsemium: For flu-like symptoms, fatigue, and weakness.

11. Bryonia: Helpful for dry coughs and headaches aggravated by movement.

12. Hepar Sulphuris: For lingering coughs and sore throats.

13. Ipecacuanha: Relieves nausea and vomiting, especially if accompanied by a clean tongue.

14. Antimonium Tartaricum: Useful for wet coughs where mucus is difficult to expel.

15. Lycopodium: Assists with digestive bloating and anxiety in shy or fearful children.

16. Rhus Toxicodendron: For joint pain and rashes, including chickenpox or poison ivy.

17. Sulphur: For skin irritations, rashes, and itchiness.

18. Apis Mellifica: Soothes insect stings and swelling.

19. Calendula: Promotes healing for cuts and minor wounds.

20. Arsenicum Album: Effective for food poisoning, diarrhea, and anxiety.

21. **Natrum Muriaticum**: Helps with colds, runny nose, and emotional stress.

22. **Carbo Vegetabilis**: Used for digestive issues, bloating, and faintness.

23. **Thuja**: Supports recovery from vaccinations or skin conditions like warts.

24. **Kali Bichromicum**: Useful for thick, stringy nasal discharge and sinus congestion.

25. **Hypericum**: Known as "Arnica for the nerves," helpful for nerve pain and injuries.

How to Administer Homeopathic Remedies

Homeopathic remedies are typically administered in pellet form, which is easy for children to take. Just a few pellets dissolved under the tongue or in water can provide relief. Because homeopathy works on an energetic level, the remedies are safe even for newborns, making it an ideal solution for parents looking for a gentle approach to healthcare.

By understanding and using the Materia Medica and Repertory, parents can feel more confident in choosing remedies that align with their child's specific symptoms, ensuring a tailored and effective approach to holistic wellness.

Acupressure for Kids: First Aid Points and How to Use Them

Acupressure is an ancient healing technique that involves applying gentle pressure to specific points on the body to promote healing and relieve discomfort. It is a simple, non-invasive way to help children manage common issues like headaches, stomachaches, or anxiety. By applying pressure to these points, you can stimulate the body's natural healing abilities.

Benefits of Acupressure for Kids

- **Non-Invasive**: No needles are used, making it child-friendly.
- **Relieves Common Discomforts**: Helps with headaches, digestion, colds, anxiety, and more.
- **Easy to Learn**: Parents can use it at home to provide quick relief.

How to Use Acupressure

To practice acupressure, use your fingertips to apply gentle, steady pressure to the points listed below. Hold the pressure for 30 seconds to 1 minute, repeating as needed. You can also gently massage the area in a circular motion.

Common Acupressure Points and Their Uses

1. LI4 (Hegu) – For Headaches and Pain Relief

- **Location**: The fleshy area between the thumb and index finger.
- **Uses**: Relieves headaches, toothaches, and general pain.

- **How to Use**: Apply gentle pressure with your thumb on one hand while supporting the hand with the other. Hold for 30-60 seconds and switch hands. Do not use during pregnancy.

2. PC6 (Neiguan) – For Nausea, Vomiting, and Anxiety

- **Location**: On the inner forearm, about three finger-widths below the wrist crease.
- **Uses**: Helps with nausea, motion sickness, upset stomach, and anxiety.
- **How to Use**: Apply steady pressure to the point using your thumb. This is especially helpful for car sickness or travel anxiety.

3. ST36 (Zusanli) – For Digestive Issues and Energy

- **Location**: Four finger-widths down from the bottom of the kneecap, along the shinbone.
- **Uses**: Improves digestion, boosts energy, and strengthens immunity.
- **How to Use**: Gently press and massage in a circular motion. This can help relieve stomachaches, constipation, or indigestion.

4. GV20 (Baihui) – For Calming and Focus

- **Location**: The top of the head, in line with the ears, where the skull meets the crown.
- **Uses**: Calms the mind, improves concentration, and helps with insomnia.
- **How to Use**: Apply gentle pressure or tap lightly on this

point to help your child relax or refocus when they are overstimulated or anxious.

5. SP6 (Sanyinjiao) – For Abdominal Pain and Sleep Issues

- **Location**: Four finger-widths above the inner ankle bone.
- **Uses**: Eases abdominal pain, regulates digestion, and promotes restful sleep.
- **How to Use**: Gently press and massage both sides of the body, applying firm but gentle pressure for 30-60 seconds.

6. BL2 (Zanzhu) – For Sinus and Allergy Relief

- **Location**: At the inner corners of the eyebrows.
- **Uses**: Helps relieve sinus congestion, headaches, and allergies.
- **How to Use**: Apply gentle pressure to both sides simultaneously, holding for up to one minute. This is effective for sinus issues or headaches due to colds.

7. LV3 (Taichong) – For Stress and Irritability

- **Location**: On the top of the foot, between the big toe and the second toe, about an inch above where the toes meet.
- **Uses**: Relieves stress, irritability, and anxiety.
- **How to Use**: Apply firm pressure to the point and massage gently for a minute. It's great for calming a child who feels overwhelmed or stressed.

8. HT7 (Shenmen) – For Emotional Balance and Restless Sleep

- **Location**: On the inner wrist, at the crease where the pinky finger side of the hand meets the wrist.
- **Uses**: Helps with emotional regulation, calming anxiety, and promoting sleep.
- **How to Use**: Gently press and hold the point for 30-60 seconds to help your child unwind or when they feel emotionally distressed.

9. UB40 (Weizhong) – For Back Pain and Muscle Tension

- **Location**: The midpoint behind the knee, in the crease.
- **Uses**: Relieves lower back pain, leg cramps, and muscle tension.
- **How to Use**: Apply gentle pressure for one minute to relieve tension in the back and legs.

10. Yintang (Third Eye Point) – For Anxiety and Insomnia

- **Location**: Midway between the eyebrows, on the forehead.
- **Uses**: Calms anxiety, promotes sleep, and relieves headaches.
- **How to Use**: Gently press or rub in circular motions for 30 seconds to a minute. This point is especially helpful for calming a child before bedtime.

Safety Guidelines for Using Acupressure with Kids

- **Gentle Pressure**: Children are sensitive, so use lighter pressure than you would on an adult. Adjust based on your child's response.
- **Monitor Reactions**: If your child feels discomfort or irrita-

tion, stop the acupressure.

- **Avoid During Illness**: Do not apply acupressure to children who are seriously ill or injured without consulting a health-care professional.
- **Do Not Use During Pregnancy**: Certain acupressure points, like LI4, should not be used during pregnancy as they can stimulate labor.

How to Integrate Acupressure Into Daily Life

Acupressure can easily become a part of your daily routine with your children. Use it as a quick remedy for common ailments or as part of a calming bedtime ritual. Teach older kids to apply gentle pressure to themselves when they're feeling anxious or out of balance.

Acupressure offers a gentle, effective way to support your child's well-being by stimulating the body's natural healing processes. Whether dealing with a minor ailment or providing a calming moment during a stressful day, these points can offer quick relief and connection.

Reflexology for Kids: A Quick Guide

Reflexology is a wonderful tool for parents who want to support their child's overall health and well-being in a gentle and soothing way. By stimulating specific points on the feet and hands, you can help relieve tension, improve circulation, and encourage the body to function optimally. Reflexology is particularly effective for children because it's calming, simple, and can help with common issues like digestive discomfort, anxiety, and sleep disturbances.

How Reflexology Works

Reflexology operates on the principle that specific points on the feet and hands correspond to different organs, glands, and body systems. By gently massaging or pressing these points, you can help stimulate the body's natural healing processes.

For children, reflexology is a calming practice that can be integrated into bedtime routines, during quiet time, or when your child is feeling unwell.

Key Reflexology Points for Kids

1. Head and Brain

- **Location**: The tips of the toes (primarily the big toe).
- **Uses**: Helps with headaches, focus, and mental clarity.
- **How to Use**: Gently press and massage the tip of the big toe for 30 seconds to 1 minute. This is great for helping kids relax and improve concentration.

2. Sinus and Nose

- **Location**: The pads of the toes (beneath the toenails).
- **Uses**: Relieves sinus pressure, colds, and congestion.
- **How to Use**: Apply gentle pressure to each toe pad, particularly during cold and flu season.

3. Lungs

- **Location**: The balls of the feet.
- **Uses**: Supports respiratory health, helps with coughs and

colds.

- **How to Use**: Use your thumbs to gently massage the balls of the feet, applying even pressure for 1-2 minutes.

4. Stomach and Digestive System

- **Location**: The arch of the foot.
- **Uses**: Helps with indigestion, constipation, and upset stomach.
- **How to Use**: Press and massage the arch of the foot in circular motions, particularly after meals to promote digestion.

5. Bladder and Kidneys

- **Location**: The middle of the foot, near the heel.
- **Uses**: Promotes healthy kidney and bladder function, helps with bedwetting and urinary issues.
- **How to Use**: Apply light pressure and massage the area just above the heel, on both feet.

6. Lower Back and Spine

- **Location**: The inner edges of the feet, running from the heel to the big toe.
- **Uses**: Helps with back pain, posture, and tension.
- **How to Use**: Massage along the inner edge of the foot, focusing on areas that may be tight or tender.

7. Solar Plexus (Calming Point)

- **Location**: The center of the foot, just below the ball.

- **Uses**: Reduces anxiety, calms nerves, promotes deep breathing.
- **How to Use**: Press gently on the center of the foot and hold for 30-60 seconds, encouraging your child to take slow, deep breaths. This point is great for bedtime or when they feel overwhelmed.

How to Use Reflexology with Kids

- **Gentle Touch**: Use a light, soothing touch when working with children. Reflexology should never be painful or uncomfortable.
- **Keep it Short**: Kids may not have the patience for long sessions, so focus on 2-3 key points for about 5-10 minutes.
- **Incorporate into Routines**: Reflexology can be a great addition to your child's bedtime or quiet time routine. It helps calm their nervous system and promotes relaxation.

Safety Tips

- **Avoid Pressure on Injured Areas**: Do not apply reflexology to areas with open wounds, fractures, or severe swelling.
- **Monitor Responses**: If your child experiences discomfort or seems unsettled, stop and adjust the pressure.

Reflexology offers a simple and effective way to support your child's health by focusing on specific pressure points that correspond to various body systems. It's a calming, holistic approach that can help with relaxation, digestion, and respiratory health.

Guide to 25 Childhood Illnesses and Holistic Remedies

1. Common Cold

- **Symptoms**: Runny nose, cough, congestion, low-grade fever.
- **Holistic Remedies**:
- **Elderberry syrup**: Supports the immune system and shortens the duration of colds.
- **Honey** (for children over 1 year): Soothes sore throats and suppresses coughing.
- **Steam inhalation**: Add eucalyptus or lavender oil to a steamy room to relieve congestion.

2. Fever

- **Symptoms**: Elevated body temperature, fatigue, body aches.
- **Holistic Remedies**:
- **Hydration**: Ensure your child drinks plenty of water, herbal teas, or diluted fruit juices.
- **Cool cloths**: Apply to the forehead, wrists, and feet to gently reduce fever.
- **Herbal baths**: Use lukewarm water with chamomile or lavender to relax and soothe your child.

3. Ear Infections

- **Symptoms**: Ear pain, fever, difficulty hearing.

- **Holistic Remedies**:
- **Garlic oil**: Warm garlic-infused olive oil and place a few drops in the ear to reduce pain and fight infection.
- **Onion compress**: A warm onion placed behind the ear can help alleviate pain.
- **Probiotics**: Boost immunity and prevent recurrent infections.

4. Sore Throat

- **Symptoms**: Painful, scratchy throat, difficulty swallowing.
- **Holistic Remedies**:
- **Saltwater gargle**: Helps reduce inflammation and kill bacteria.
- **Herbal teas**: Chamomile and slippery elm tea soothe the throat.
- **Honey and lemon**: Combine for a throat-soothing remedy.

5. Cough

- **Symptoms**: Dry or productive cough.
- **Holistic Remedies**:
- **Thyme tea**: A natural cough suppressant that relaxes the bronchial muscles.
- **Honey and cinnamon**: Mix to help soothe a cough.
- **Steam therapy**: Add eucalyptus oil to a bowl of hot water and have your child inhale the steam.

6. Constipation

- **Symptoms**: Difficulty passing stools, abdominal pain.

- **Holistic Remedies**:
- **Increase fiber**: Give prunes, pears, and apples to encourage regularity.
- **Flaxseed oil**: A gentle laxative that supports digestive health.
- **Massage**: Gently massage the abdomen in a clockwise motion to stimulate digestion.

7. Diarrhea

- **Symptoms**: Loose, watery stools, stomach cramping.
- **Holistic Remedies**:
- **Bananas, rice, applesauce, and toast (BRAT diet)**: Soothes the stomach and helps bind stools.
- **Probiotics**: Help restore gut flora and shorten the duration of diarrhea.
- **Chamomile tea**: Soothes the stomach and reduces inflammation.

8. Colic

- **Symptoms**: Prolonged crying, discomfort, gassiness.
- **Holistic Remedies**:
- **Gripe water**: A blend of herbs like fennel and ginger that helps reduce gas.
- **Infant massage**: Gently rub the baby's belly in a clockwise motion to relieve gas.
- **Chamomile tea** (for breastfeeding moms): Passed through breast milk to calm the baby's digestive system.

9. Teething

- **Symptoms**: Drooling, irritability, swollen gums.
- **Holistic Remedies**:
- **Cold washcloth**: Let your baby chew on a cold, damp washcloth to soothe gums.
- **Chamomile tea**: Rub a few drops on the gums to calm irritation.
- **Amber teething necklace**: Believed to help reduce inflammation and pain.

10. Eczema

- **Symptoms**: Dry, itchy, inflamed skin.
- **Holistic Remedies**:
- **Coconut oil**: Moisturizes and soothes irritated skin.
- **Oatmeal baths**: Reduces itching and inflammation.
- **Calendula cream**: Heals and protects dry skin.

11. Chickenpox

- **Symptoms**: Itchy rash, fever, fatigue.
- **Holistic Remedies**:
- **Oatmeal baths**: Relieves itching and soothes the skin.
- **Calendula**: Apply calendula cream to reduce itching and inflammation.
- **Baking soda paste**: Mix with water to apply to itchy spots.

12. Hand, Foot, and Mouth Disease

- **Symptoms**: Fever, mouth sores, rash on hands and feet.
- **Holistic Remedies**:
- **Coconut water**: Keeps your child hydrated and soothes

mouth sores.

- **Calendula cream**: Soothes and heals rashes.
- **Chamomile tea**: Helps reduce fever and calm irritation.

13. Asthma

- **Symptoms**: Wheezing, shortness of breath, coughing.
- **Holistic Remedies**:
- **Steam inhalation**: Helps open airways and reduce inflammation.
- **Magnesium-rich foods**: Magnesium helps relax bronchial muscles.
- **Avoid triggers**: Identify and avoid allergens like dust and pet dander.

14. Seasonal Allergies

- **Symptoms**: Runny nose, sneezing, itchy eyes.
- **Holistic Remedies**:
- **Local honey**: Consuming local honey may help reduce pollen sensitivity.
- **Nettle tea**: Acts as a natural antihistamine.
- **Saline nasal spray**: Clears allergens from the nasal passages.

15. Earwax Buildup

- **Symptoms**: Ear discomfort, trouble hearing, earache.
- **Holistic Remedies**:
- **Warm olive oil**: A few drops in the ear can soften earwax for easier removal.

- **Hydrogen peroxide**: Mix with water and place a few drops in the ear to break down wax.
- **Massage**: Gently massage the area around the ear to help loosen wax.

16. Croup

- **Symptoms**: Barking cough, difficulty breathing, hoarseness.
- **Holistic Remedies**:
- **Steam therapy**: Run a hot shower and let your child breathe in the steam.
- **Cool mist humidifier**: Helps soothe the airway and ease breathing.
- **Honey** (for children over 1 year): Soothes the throat and reduces coughing.

17. Cradle Cap

- **Symptoms**: Yellow, crusty patches on a baby's scalp.
- **Holistic Remedies**:
- **Coconut oil**: Gently massage into the scalp and brush out flakes.
- **Olive oil**: Softens the patches for easy removal.
- **Calendula**: Apply a small amount to soothe and moisturize the scalp.

18. Pink Eye (Conjunctivitis)

- **Symptoms**: Red, itchy eyes, discharge.
- **Holistic Remedies**:

- **Breast milk**: Apply a few drops to the eye to help fight infection.
- **Chamomile tea compress**: Soothes irritation and reduces inflammation.
- **Honey and water rinse**: A natural antibacterial solution for washing the eye.

19. Growing Pains

- **Symptoms**: Leg aches, particularly at night.
- **Holistic Remedies**:
- **Epsom salt baths**: Relaxes muscles and eases pain.
- **Magnesium lotion**: Massage into the legs to reduce pain.
- **Warm compress**: Place on the affected area to soothe soreness.

20. Hives

- **Symptoms**: Itchy, raised welts on the skin.
- **Holistic Remedies**:
- **Oatmeal baths**: Relieves itching and soothes irritation.
- **Cold compresses**: Reduce swelling and itching.
- **Calendula cream**: Apply to hives to reduce inflammation.

21. Warts

- **Symptoms**: Small, rough skin growths.
- **Holistic Remedies**:
- **Apple cider vinegar**: Apply with a cotton ball and cover with a bandage.
- **Banana peel**: Tape the inside of a banana peel to the wart

overnight.

- **Tea tree oil**: Dab a small amount onto the wart daily.

22. Ringworm

- **Symptoms**: Circular rash with a raised, red border.
- **Holistic Remedies**:
- **Coconut oil**: Antifungal properties help heal ringworm.
- **Tea tree oil**: Apply diluted tea tree oil to the rash.
- **Aloe vera**: Soothes itching and promotes healing.

23. Hand Eczema

- **Symptoms**: Dry, cracked skin on hands.
- **Holistic Remedies**:
- **Shea butter**: Moisturizes and soothes the skin.
- **Oatmeal baths**: Reduces itching and inflammation.
- **Calendula**: Heals and protects dry, cracked skin.

24. Nosebleeds

- **Symptoms**: Bleeding from the nose.
- **Holistic Remedies**:
- **Saline spray**: Moisturizes dry nasal passages to prevent bleeding.
- **Cold compress**: Apply to the nose to stop the bleeding.
- **Humidifier**: Keeps the air moist and prevents nasal dryness.

25. Bruises

- **Symptoms**: Skin discoloration and swelling from an impact.

- **Holistic Remedies**:
- **Arnica cream**: Reduces swelling and promotes healing.
- **Cold compress**: Apply to the bruise to reduce swelling.
- **Witch hazel**: Soothes and reduces bruising.

Holistic remedies can support your child's healing process while addressing symptoms naturally and gently. These remedies can be easily incorporated into daily care routines, empowering you as a mother to provide comfort and relief at home.

Holistic Medicine Cabinet Essentials for Mamas

1. Elderberry Syrup

- **Uses**: Boosts immune function, shortens the duration of colds and flu.
- **Why Keep It**: Elderberry syrup is a go-to remedy for immune support during cold and flu season.

2. Honey (Raw, Unprocessed)

- **Uses**: Soothes coughs and sore throats, acts as a natural antibacterial.
- **Why Keep It**: Honey is excellent for coughs, burns, and minor cuts (for children over 1 year).

3. Coconut Oil

- **Uses**: Skin moisturizer, helps with diaper rash, minor cuts, and scrapes.

- **Why Keep It**: Coconut oil has antimicrobial properties and is a versatile remedy for the skin and digestive health.

4. Arnica Cream or Gel

- **Uses**: Reduces bruising, muscle pain, and inflammation.
- **Why Keep It**: Arnica is ideal for treating bumps, bruises, and sore muscles after physical activity.

5. Calendula Cream

- **Uses**: Heals minor burns, cuts, scrapes, and rashes.
- **Why Keep It**: A gentle cream for skin irritations, safe for children with sensitive skin.

6. Probiotics

- **Uses**: Supports gut health, helps with constipation, diarrhea, and immune support.
- **Why Keep It**: Probiotics help maintain a healthy digestive system and boost immunity, especially after antibiotics.

7. Activated Charcoal

- **Uses**: Treats mild food poisoning, gas, and bloating.
- **Why Keep It**: Useful for stomach upsets and digestive issues, helping to eliminate toxins from the body.

8. Chamomile Tea or Tincture

- **Uses**: Soothes digestive issues, calms anxiety, helps with teething.
- **Why Keep It**: Chamomile is gentle and effective for calming children and helping with sleep or upset stomachs.

9. Lavender Essential Oil

- **Uses**: Promotes relaxation, calms anxiety, helps with sleep, and soothes minor burns.
- **Why Keep It**: A must-have for bedtime routines, minor skin irritations, and calming anxiety.

10. Peppermint Essential Oil

- **Uses**: Relieves headaches, digestive upset, and congestion.
- **Why Keep It**: A versatile oil for tummy troubles, headaches, or adding to steam inhalation for colds.

11. Epsom Salt

- **Uses**: Relieves muscle tension, detoxifies, and soothes skin irritations.
- **Why Keep It**: Great for warm baths to relax muscles, reduce stress, or treat skin irritations like eczema.

12. Gripe Water

- **Uses**: Relieves colic, gas, and upset stomachs in infants.
- **Why Keep It**: A safe, natural remedy for newborns with digestive discomfort.

13. Witch Hazel

- **Uses**: Soothes insect bites, reduces bruising, and acts as an astringent for minor cuts.
- **Why Keep It**: A natural remedy for swelling, bites, and minor scrapes.

14. Oregano Oil (Diluted)

- **Uses**: Antibacterial, antiviral, and supports immune function.
- **Why Keep It**: Oregano oil is a potent natural remedy for fighting infections.

15. Rescue Remedy (Bach Flower Blend)

- **Uses**: Eases anxiety, stress, and emotional upset.
- **Why Keep It**: Great for calming emotional distress in kids during stressful situations, such as doctor visits or school exams.

16. Homeopathic Arnica Pellets

- **Uses**: Reduces swelling, bruising, and muscle pain.
- **Why Keep It**: Easy to administer and effective for treating minor injuries and trauma.

17. Zinc Lozenges

- **Uses**: Boosts the immune system and reduces the duration of colds.

- **Why Keep It**: Zinc supports recovery from colds and sore throats, and is helpful during the winter months.

18. **Colloidal Silver**

- **Uses**: Antibacterial, antiviral, can be used topically for cuts or taken orally for infections.
- **Why Keep It**: Colloidal silver is a natural antibiotic alternative for minor infections.

19. **Aloe Vera Gel**

- **Uses**: Soothes sunburns, skin irritations, and cuts.
- **Why Keep It**: A cooling gel that is perfect for burns, rashes, and other skin irritations.

20. **Hydrogen Peroxide (3%)**

- **Uses**: Cleans wounds and helps with ear infections.
- **Why Keep It**: A basic first-aid antiseptic for cleaning wounds and ear irrigation.

21. **Castor Oil**

- **Uses**: Stimulates bowel movements and helps with skin conditions.
- **Why Keep It**: A safe, gentle laxative for constipation, also useful for skin and hair care.

22. **Bentonite Clay**

- **Uses**: Detoxifies the skin, treats bites, stings, and mild burns.
- **Why Keep It**: An effective natural detoxifier that draws toxins out of the skin when used as a poultice.

23. Slippery Elm

- **Uses**: Soothes sore throats, digestive upset, and helps with colds.
- **Why Keep It**: A gentle herb that helps with coughs, sore throats, and gastrointestinal issues.

24. Apple Cider Vinegar

- **Uses**: Balances pH, helps with digestion, and soothes sore throats.
- **Why Keep It**: Great for balancing internal health, and can be used topically for skin irritations.

25. Magnesium Lotion

- **Uses**: Relieves muscle cramps, growing pains, and promotes relaxation.
- **Why Keep It**: Magnesium is essential for muscle function and can help calm restless kids at bedtime.

Key Tools to Keep in Your Holistic Medicine Cabinet

- **Thermometer**: For checking fever accurately.
- **Humidifier**: Helps ease respiratory issues, congestion, and dry skin.

- **Hot/Cold Compress**: Great for reducing swelling, fevers, and soothing aches.
- **Neti Pot**: For nasal irrigation, clearing congestion naturally.
- **Essential Oil Diffuser**: To diffuse oils for relaxation, congestion, or immune support.

By stocking your holistic medicine cabinet with these natural remedies and tools, you'll be prepared to handle a wide variety of common childhood ailments naturally. These items allow you to treat minor illnesses, support immunity, and provide comfort to your family, all while maintaining a gentle, holistic approach to health.

When to Use Natural Remedies vs. Conventional Medicine

Knowing When to Seek Medical Help

While natural remedies can be highly effective for many common ailments, there are times when conventional medicine is necessary. It's important to know the difference between a condition that can be managed with herbs and oils and one that requires a doctor's attention. Here are a few guidelines:

- **Fevers Over 103°F**: If your child's fever climbs over 103°F and doesn't respond to natural remedies like cool baths or herbal teas, it's time to seek medical advice.
- **Persistent Symptoms**: If symptoms persist for more than a few days or worsen, despite the use of natural remedies, a medical evaluation may be necessary to rule out more serious conditions.
- **Breathing Difficulties**: Any sign of difficulty breathing, wheezing, or prolonged coughing should be addressed by a healthcare professional immediately.

Understanding when to integrate conventional medicine ensures that you're not taking unnecessary risks with your child's health, while still benefiting from the gentler options that natural remedies provide.

Empowering Parents to Make Health Decisions

When parents are knowledgeable about natural remedies, they feel empowered to make informed decisions for their child's health. By understanding the strengths and limitations of natural remedies, you can confidently care for your child at home while staying mindful of when to seek outside help. This balance between holistic and conventional medicine is key to raising a healthy, well-balanced child.

Wesley's Ear Infections and the Onion Poultice Miracle

I always took pride in how healthy Wesley was, rarely getting sick even as a toddler. But that all changed when he started daycare at 21 months. Suddenly, Wesley faced a series of challenges, and before I knew it, he had developed three ear infections back to back. We tried two rounds of antibiotics, hoping they would help him recover, but the infections kept returning. Desperation led me to explore alternative solutions.

That's when I remembered an old remedy I had read about: an onion poultice. With a mixture of doubt and hope, I sent my boyfriend to the store for a yellow onion. I baked it at 400 degrees for 25 minutes, and once it was warm but not scalding, I held it gently over Wesley's ear. Some sources suggested squeezing the onion juice directly into the ear, but I decided not to take that step.

To my surprise and relief, the simple onion poultice worked wonders. Wesley's ear infection eased, and he slept through the night for the first time in days. That moment reinforced my belief in the power of natural remedies and how sometimes, the simplest solutions can have profound effects.

A Household's Transition to Herbal Remedies

The Williams family once relied heavily on over-the-counter medications for everything from colds to headaches. But after their youngest child developed recurring ear infections, they began to question whether the constant use of antibiotics and medications was necessary. With the guidance of a holistic health practitioner, they slowly transitioned to using herbal remedies. They introduced echinacea tea for colds, elderberry syrup to boost immunity, and garlic oil to relieve ear infections naturally. Over time, they noticed that their children's overall health improved, and the need for frequent doctor visits decreased. This shift in approach gave the family a new sense of control over their health, and they now keep a fully stocked herbal medicine cabinet.

A Mother's Journey into Herbal Medicine

Sarah, a mother of three, became interested in natural remedies when her second child was born with severe eczema. After trying countless creams and medications with little success, she began researching herbal remedies that might offer relief. She found that calendula and chamomile creams helped soothe her son's irritated skin, and dietary changes to support gut health also played a key role. Inspired by the results, Sarah enrolled in an herbal medicine course and began sharing her newfound knowledge with friends and family. Now, she leads workshops in her community, teaching other parents how to integrate natural remedies into their family's healthcare routines.

Natural remedies empower families to address common health issues safely and effectively. By learning to use herbs, essential oils, tinctures, and homeopathy, parents can provide gentle, holistic care for their children while avoiding the overuse of conventional medications. These remedies align with a holistic approach to wellness, offering natural relief for everyday ailments.

By incorporating natural remedies into your family's health routine, you deepen your commitment to holistic health practices. This approach not only promotes healing but also empowers you to take control of your child's health, offering natural relief from everyday ailments.

In the next chapter, we will address a modern challenge that many families face: balancing screen time with outdoor play and natural experiences. We'll explore strategies for creating a healthy balance between technology and nature, supporting your child's physical and emotional well-being.

11

Balancing Screen Time and Green Time

In today's digital age, technology is everywhere—at home, at school, and in the hands of our children. While screens offer convenience and entertainment, the challenge for parents is finding the right balance between the virtual world and real-world experiences. Excessive screen time can negatively impact a child's development, while outdoor play provides numerous physical, emotional, and cognitive benefits. As parents, it's essential to foster a healthy relationship with technology while encouraging children to engage with the natural world around them.

Striking a balance between screen time and "green time" is critical for supporting healthy development in children. While screens have their place, spending time outdoors fosters creativity, emotional resilience, and cognitive development. In this chapter, we'll explore the effects of screen time, the benefits of outdoor play, and practical strategies for creating a balanced, tech-healthy lifestyle for your family.

The Effects of Screen Time

Cognitive and Emotional Impact

Excessive screen time can have a significant impact on a child's cognitive development and emotional regulation. Research has shown that too much screen exposure, especially during critical developmental years, can affect a child's attention span, behavior, and ability to manage emotions. Fast-paced, highly stimulating digital content can make it harder for children to focus on tasks that require sustained attention, like reading or problem-solving. Moreover, when screen time replaces real-world interactions, children may struggle with social skills and emotional regulation, as screens don't provide the same opportunities for learning empathy, communication, and conflict resolution.

Physical Consequences

Beyond the cognitive and emotional effects, too much screen time can take a toll on a child's physical health. Hours spent sitting in front of a screen contribute to poor posture, eye strain, and even childhood obesity. Children who spend a significant amount of time on devices are less likely to engage in physical activity, leading to a sedentary lifestyle that can have long-term health implications. Encouraging "green time"—time spent outdoors in active play—helps counterbalance the physical downsides of excessive screen use.

Encouraging Outdoor Play

The Benefits of Nature

Nature is a powerful antidote to the overstimulation that screens often provide. Time spent in green spaces—whether it's a local park, a forest hike, or simply playing in the backyard—offers a wide range of benefits for children. Studies show that time outdoors improves mood, reduces stress, and enhances creativity. Exposure to nature also supports cognitive function, helping children focus better and solve problems more effectively.

Outdoor play fosters independence and creativity, allowing children to explore their environment, take risks, and engage in imaginative play. It also provides opportunities for social interaction, whether through cooperative games, team sports, or unstructured play with friends. These experiences are essential for emotional resilience, helping children develop confidence, social skills, and the ability to navigate challenges in the real world.

Strategies for Promoting Outdoor Activities

Getting kids excited about spending time outside can sometimes be challenging, especially when screens seem more appealing. Here are a few creative strategies to encourage outdoor play:

- **Nature Scavenger Hunts**: Create a list of natural objects (like leaves, rocks, or flowers) for your child to find on a walk or in the backyard. It adds an element of adventure and makes exploring nature more engaging.
- **Gardening Projects**: Involve your child in planting a garden or caring for a small herb pot. Gardening teaches responsibility and connects children to the cycles of nature.
- **Outdoor Art**: Set up an outdoor art station where your child can paint, draw, or create nature-inspired crafts. Using natural materials like leaves or stones can spark creativity and encourage exploration.
- **Family Hikes or Bike Rides**: Make outdoor activities a family event by going on hikes, nature walks, or bike rides together. It's a great way to bond while being active and enjoying the fresh air.

These simple activities can help shift your child's focus from the screen to the wonders of the natural world, offering a balanced, holistic approach to play.

Establishing Healthy Tech Boundaries

Family Guidelines for Technology Use

Creating clear guidelines for technology use in the household is essential for maintaining a healthy balance between screen time and outdoor play. Here are some strategies to set tech boundaries in your home:

- **Tech-Free Zones**: Designate certain areas of your home, like the dining room or bedrooms, as tech-free zones. This encourages face-to-face interaction and helps create spaces for relaxation without digital distractions.
- **Tech-Free Times**: Establish tech-free times during the day, such as family mealtimes or the hour before bed. These moments provide an opportunity for meaningful conversation and help children wind down before sleep.
- **Screen Time Limits**: Set daily or weekly limits on screen time, depending on your child's age and needs. Encourage your child to spend the majority of their free time engaging in outdoor play, reading, or creative activities instead of in front of a screen.

Leading by Example

Children are more likely to adopt healthy tech habits if they see their parents modeling the same behaviors. As parents, it's important to be mindful of your own screen use and to prioritize spending time outdoors as a family. Whether it's going for a walk, playing a sport, or simply enjoying a picnic in the park, making outdoor activities part of your family's routine reinforces the value of "green time." By leading by example, you show your children that life outside the screen is rich with experiences, learning, and connection.

Embracing Nature's Benefits

Incorporating outdoor activities in state and national parks, local parks, hiking trails, and camping grounds is essential for a balanced lifestyle. Programs like *1000 Hours Outside* encourage families to spend time outdoors, promoting physical activity, creativity, and connection with nature. These green zones are not just spaces for play; they help reduce stress, foster resilience, and build healthier relationships.

When planning outdoor activities, consider local parks for regular play, weekend camping trips to state parks, or even exploring nearby national parks for a more immersive experience. Hiking together or having picnics reinforces the joy of movement and exploration. Balancing time in these natural environments with mindful screen use helps establish a healthy routine that supports physical and emotional development for children.

A Humorous Story About a Family's Tech-Free Weekend

One weekend, the Johnson family decided to go completely tech-free—no phones, no tablets, no TV. At first, the kids were horrified, asking, "But what will we do all day?" But as the weekend unfolded, something surprising happened. Without screens to distract them, the children got creative. They built forts out of blankets, made up games in the backyard, and even invented a "family Olympics" with obstacle courses and races. The parents were amazed at the imaginative play that emerged once the screens were off. By Sunday evening, the kids admitted,

"That was actually kind of fun!" It was a reminder that when given the chance, children are naturally creative and resourceful, and they don't need screens to be entertained.

Family Success Stories of Reducing Screen Time

The Thompson family was concerned that their two boys were spending too much time on their tablets, becoming irritable and disengaged. They decided to adopt screen-free weekdays, allowing limited screen time only on weekends. At first, the boys resisted, but after a few weeks, their behavior began to change. They became more active, spending hours outdoors riding bikes, playing basketball, and even reading more. Their focus improved, and their creativity flourished as they found new ways to play and interact with each other. The family noticed a positive shift in mood and energy levels, proving that less screen time led to more engaged, happier children.

Balancing screen time with outdoor "green time" is essential for fostering healthy development in children. Time spent outdoors not only supports physical health but also enhances social skills, creativity, and emotional well-being. By creating healthy boundaries around technology use and encouraging outdoor activities, parents can help their children develop a balanced relationship with screens and the natural world.

This chapter emphasizes the importance of finding equilibrium between technology and nature. By supporting your child's natural growth through outdoor play, you're fostering their physical, emotional, and cognitive development while helping them manage the digital distractions of the modern world.

Next, we'll explore the role of emotional wellness in early childhood development. We'll discuss how to nurture emotional intelligence, build resilience, and support your child's ability to manage stress and emotions.

12

Emotional Wellness in Early Development

Imagine the peace and calm of a serene garden. In the midst of life's busyness, we all need that sense of stillness and inner peace—especially children. Just as physical health is essential for a child's development, emotional wellness is equally critical. Cultivating emotional resilience and inner calm in children is key to raising well-balanced, emotionally healthy individuals who can thrive in a complex world. This chapter explores the importance of emotional wellness, providing strategies to help children manage stress, express their emotions healthily, and build emotional resilience.

Emotional wellness is a vital component of holistic health, helping children learn to navigate stress, build resilience, and express their emotions in healthy ways. Supporting a child's emotional development lays the foundation for them to grow into confident, emotionally balanced adults. In this chapter, we'll explore how to nurture emotional intelligence and build resilience from an early age.

Nurturing Emotional Intelligence

Recognizing and Addressing Emotions

Teaching children to recognize and express their emotions is the first step in building emotional intelligence. Emotional literacy begins with helping children identify what they're feeling—whether it's joy, frustration, sadness, or excitement. Naming emotions gives children the language they need to express themselves, which is crucial for their emotional and social development.

Parents can create safe spaces for children to talk about their feelings, whether it's after a tough day at school or when they're feeling anxious about a new experience. Validating their emotions, rather than dismissing them, helps children understand that all feelings are normal and can be managed healthily. Simple conversations like, "It seems like you're feeling frustrated—can you tell me why?" allow children to start recognizing and processing their emotions rather than bottling them up.

Mindfulness and Meditation for Kids

Mindfulness practices can help children develop focus, manage stress, and cultivate inner peace. Teaching children simple mindfulness exercises, such as deep breathing or guided meditation, gives them tools to calm their minds in stressful situations.

For younger children, mindfulness can be as simple as teaching them to focus on their breathing by imagining their belly is a balloon inflating and deflating. For older children, guided meditations or visualizations can help them unwind and relax. These practices not only help in the moment but also build lifelong skills in stress management and emotional regulation.

Incorporating mindfulness into daily routines—whether it's taking a few minutes to breathe deeply before bed or practicing mindful eating during meals—helps children connect with their emotions and stay grounded in the present moment.

Building Emotional Resilience

The Power of Positive Reinforcement

Positive reinforcement plays a powerful role in building emotional resilience in children. When children are encouraged and praised for their efforts, they develop self-esteem and emotional strength. This isn't about empty praise but about recognizing and celebrating their achievements, big or small. Positive reinforcement can take many forms, from verbal encouragement to rewards like extra playtime.

Praising a child's problem-solving abilities, for example, fosters confidence in their capacity to handle challenges. "You worked so hard on that puzzle, and even though it was tough, you didn't give up!" reinforces the idea that perseverance and effort are more important than instant success. This type of feedback helps children build the resilience they'll need to face life's inevitable difficulties.

Teaching Problem-Solving Skills

Life will always present challenges, and one of the most important skills children can learn is how to navigate conflict and problem-solve. Teaching children to approach problems with a calm mind and creative solutions helps them become emotionally resilient.

Guided problem-solving involves walking through challenges together, asking open-ended questions like, "What do you think we could try to make this better?" or "How do you think we can solve this problem together?" This approach helps children think critically and explore different solutions without becoming overwhelmed by frustration or defeat. Over time, they'll begin to apply these strategies independently, developing emotional resilience that will serve them throughout life.

Mindfulness in Family Life: A Calming Transformation

Incorporating mindfulness into daily family life can have profound effects. One mother shared her experience of introducing mindfulness exercises to her son, who had been struggling with anxiety. Each night before bed, they would spend a few minutes practicing deep breathing and visualization, imagining they were in a peaceful, calming place. Over time, her son's anxiety levels decreased, and he began using these techniques independently whenever he felt stressed. What began as a small practice evolved into a valuable tool for emotional regulation that transformed their family dynamic.

A Child's Journey from Stress to Inner Peace

Another family shared their journey of helping their daughter, Emily, who had been overwhelmed by stress due to school pressures and social challenges. They began integrating mindfulness and positive reinforcement into her daily routine. Her parents would acknowledge her feelings and celebrate her small victories, helping her reframe setbacks as opportunities for growth. Through guided problem-solving and mindfulness exercises, Emily learned to manage her stress more effectively and found a sense of inner peace. By the end of the year, her teachers noticed a remarkable improvement in her focus and emotional balance.

Bach Flower Remedies: A Gentle Path to Emotional Balance

Bach Flower Remedies are a collection of 38 flower essences that support emotional and mental well-being. Developed by Dr. Edward Bach, these remedies are designed to treat the emotional and psychological roots of imbalance, promoting emotional harmony. Each remedy corresponds to a specific emotion or state of mind, making them a valuable tool for managing stress, fear, anxiety, or mood swings in children and adults alike.

The remedies are safe, non-toxic, and can be used alongside other treatments without concern for interactions. They are gentle enough for children and can be easily incorporated into daily routines.

How to Use Bach Flower Remedies

Direct Use: Add 2 drops of the selected remedy into a glass of water, and sip throughout the day.

Combination: Up to 7 remedies can be combined in a single treatment bottle. To create a combination, add 2 drops of each selected remedy to a small bottle of water and take 4 drops at regular intervals.

Topical Application: The remedies can also be applied directly to pulse points, such as the wrists or behind the ears, using a dropper or cotton pad.

For children, you can dilute the remedy further in water or juice if they are sensitive to taste as most of the time brandy or glycerin are used to preserve the flower essence.

The 38 Bach Flower Remedies and Their Uses

Agrimony - For children who hide their worries behind a brave face or humor. Helps promote emotional honesty and acceptance.

Aspen - For vague fears, nightmares, or anxiety without a clear cause. Provides a sense of safety and peace.

Beech - For intolerance and irritability. Helps children become more understanding and patient with others.

Centaury - For children who find it hard to say no, often overextending themselves. Helps them set healthy boundaries.

Cerato - For indecisiveness and lack of self-trust. Encourages confidence in one's own judgment.

Cherry Plum - For children who feel they are losing control, especially during tantrums. Promotes calm and control.

Chestnut Bud - For children who repeat the same mistakes. Enhances learning from experiences.

Chicory – For children who are overly possessive or needy. Encourages selfless love and emotional independence.

Clematis – For daydreamers and children who are inattentive or disengaged. Helps them feel more present and focused.

Crab Apple – For children who feel self-conscious or uncomfortable with their bodies. Encourages self-acceptance.

Elm – For children who feel overwhelmed by responsibility. Helps restore confidence and perspective.

Gentian – For discouragement after setbacks or failures. Encourages optimism and perseverance.

Gorse – For hopelessness and feelings of giving up. Helps foster hope and renewed motivation.

Heather – For children who feel lonely or overly talkative, craving constant attention. Encourages self-reliance.

Holly – For jealousy, envy, or sibling rivalry. Promotes love, understanding, and emotional harmony.

Honeysuckle – For children who dwell on the past or are homesick. Encourages living in the present.

Hornbeam - For mental fatigue or lack of motivation, especially when facing daily tasks. Revitalizes energy and enthusiasm.

Impatiens - For restlessness, impatience, and frustration. Helps cultivate calm and patience.

Larch - For children who lack confidence and fear failure. Promotes self-assurance and willingness to try.

Mimulus - For children who are shy or fearful of known things (e.g., animals, darkness). Helps build courage and confidence.

Mustard - For sudden sadness or low mood with no apparent cause. Encourages emotional balance and stability.

Oak - For children who work hard and take on too much but become worn out. Helps them find balance and rest.

Olive - For exhaustion after physical or emotional effort. Restores vitality and energy.

Pine - For children who feel guilty or blame themselves. Helps release feelings of guilt and promotes self-compassion.

Red Chestnut - For children who worry excessively about others, especially family members. Encourages trust and peace of mind.

Rock Rose – For panic or terror, especially after traumatic experiences. Instills courage and calm.

Rock Water – For children who are too hard on themselves and set rigid standards. Promotes flexibility and self-kindness.

Scleranthus – For indecision, especially between two choices. Helps restore inner balance and decisiveness.

Star of Bethlehem – For emotional trauma or shock. Offers comfort and healing after difficult experiences.

Sweet Chestnut – For children who feel hopeless or in despair. Encourages renewal and faith in a positive outcome.

Vervain – For children who are overly enthusiastic or have trouble winding down. Encourages relaxation and moderation.

Vine – For children who tend to be bossy or domineering. Helps foster respect and teamwork.

Walnut – For children going through big changes, like moving, a new sibling, or starting school. Offers protection and adjustment.

Water Violet – For children who are withdrawn or prefer solitude. Encourages connection and empathy.

White Chestnut – For racing thoughts, worry, or trouble falling asleep. Promotes calm and mental clarity.

Wild Oat – For indecision about life direction, particularly during adolescence. Encourages clarity of purpose.

Wild Rose – For children who appear apathetic or resigned. Promotes enthusiasm for life and engagement.

Willow – For resentment or bitterness, especially if they feel life is unfair. Encourages forgiveness and positivity.

Using Rescue Remedy

In addition to the 38 individual remedies, Rescue Remedy is a pre-blended combination of five remedies (Rock Rose, Impatiens, Clematis, Star of Bethlehem, and Cherry Plum) designed for use during moments of acute stress or crisis. It is especially useful for children during times of anxiety, such as school exams, doctor visits, or emotional upsets.

How to Use: Add 4 drops of Rescue Remedy to water or juice, or apply directly to the tongue or pulse points.

Bach Flower Remedies offer a gentle, natural way to support children's emotional health by addressing specific feelings and states of mind. They can be easily integrated into daily routines to help children feel more balanced, calm, and emotionally resilient.

Breathing Exercises for Kids: Tools for Self-Regulation and Calm

Teaching children to use simple breathing exercises can help them manage emotions, reduce stress, and develop better self-control. Breathing exercises are easy to incorporate into daily routines, and they offer a grounding tool that children can use whenever they need to calm down or refocus.

1. Cookie Breathing

How to Do It: Imagine holding a warm cookie fresh from the oven. Take a slow, deep breath in through your nose to "smell the cookies," then pause. Next, exhale slowly through your mouth as if blowing on the cookie to cool it down.

Benefits: This exercise helps children focus on their breath, grounding them and slowing their breathing. By engaging the imagination, it makes deep breathing enjoyable and accessible for kids.

Why It Works: Cookie breathing encourages self-regulation and self-control by training children to pause and calm themselves. It's particularly helpful in moments of frustration or excitement, giving them a tool to refocus.

2. Bumblebee Breathing

How to Do It: Take a deep breath in through the nose, then exhale while making a gentle "mmm" or humming sound, like a buzzing bee. (This also helps with natural production of Nitric oxide in the body.)

Benefits: The humming vibration helps to calm the nervous system and encourages children to focus on their breathing rhythm.

Why It Works: Bumblebee breathing provides sensory feedback through the hum, which can be soothing for children and helps them stay engaged with the exercise.

3. Balloon Breathing

How to Do It: Imagine you are blowing up a balloon. Take a deep breath in, then exhale slowly, pretending to fill the balloon with air. Visualize the balloon getting bigger and bigger with each exhale.

Benefits: This exercise encourages children to take deep, controlled breaths, which can reduce stress and help with concentration.

Why It Works: Visualizing the balloon filling up helps children slow down their breathing, which naturally helps to calm the body and mind.

When to Use Breathing Exercises with Kids

Breathing exercises are ideal during transitions, before bedtime, or anytime children need to calm down. Incorporating these exercises into daily routines can make them a habit, empowering children to use them independently when they need to manage emotions or focus.

Meditating with Your Kids: A Path to Calm and Connection

Introducing meditation to children can be a powerful tool for emotional regulation, focus, and relaxation. Children naturally experience stress and anxiety, whether it's from school, friendships, or daily routines, and meditation offers them a way to pause, calm their minds, and connect with their emotions in a healthy way.

Meditating with your kids not only helps them cultivate mindfulness but also creates moments of connection and bonding. It's a simple practice that can be incorporated into daily routines, whether it's during bedtime, after school, or even in moments of tension.

Benefits of Meditating with Kids

- **Emotional Regulation:** Meditation helps children recognize and manage their emotions, giving them tools to calm down when they're feeling anxious, upset, or overwhelmed.
- **Improved Focus and Concentration:** Regular meditation can improve attention and reduce distractions, which can benefit children both academically and socially.
- **Better Sleep:** Bedtime meditations can help ease children into sleep by relaxing their bodies and minds.
- **Enhanced Self-Awareness:** Meditation teaches kids to tune

into their bodies and emotions, fostering a greater sense of self-awareness and empathy.

How to Introduce Meditation to Kids

1. **Keep It Short:** Start with short sessions, especially for younger children. Even 3 to 5 minutes is a great start.
2. **Make It Fun:** Use engaging imagery, guided breathing, and playful language to keep them interested.
3. **Create a Calm Environment:** Choose a quiet, comfortable space for meditation. You can set the mood by dimming the lights or playing calming music.
4. **Lead by Example:** Meditate with your children. When they see you practicing mindfulness, they're more likely to follow along and make it a regular habit.

Meditation Scripts for Kids

Here are a few simple meditation scripts you can use with your children. These can be done anytime, but they are especially effective before bed or during moments when your child is feeling anxious or overstimulated.

1. Balloon Breathing (3-5 minutes)

This simple breathing meditation helps children calm down and focus on their breath.

Script:

"Close your eyes and imagine that you are holding a big balloon in your hands. What color is your balloon? Now, take a deep breath in through your nose, filling up your belly like you are blowing up the balloon. As you breathe out through your mouth, imagine the balloon getting bigger and bigger. Take another deep breath in, feeling your belly grow, and slowly breathe out again, making the balloon even bigger. Let's do this a few more times—inhale, blow up the balloon, and exhale, making the balloon float gently. When you're ready, let go of your balloon and watch it float away into the sky. Feel your body relaxed and calm."

2. Butterfly Relaxation (5 minutes)

This guided visualization helps children relax their bodies and minds by imagining they are a butterfly.

Script:

"Close your eyes and take a deep breath in. Now imagine that you are a butterfly. What color are your wings? Imagine yourself flying gently through a garden, floating from flower to flower. The sun is shining on your wings, and you feel the warmth of the sun. As you land on a flower, take a deep breath in, and let your body feel light and calm. Now, gently flap your wings as you fly to another flower. Feel how soft the wind is as you move. You are light, free, and peaceful. Now, slowly land on a soft petal and rest there, breathing in and out slowly. When you're ready, slowly open your eyes, bringing that calm and peaceful feeling with you."

3. Starry Night Relaxation (5-7 minutes)

This bedtime meditation helps children relax and prepare for sleep by imagining they are lying under the stars.

Script:

"Close your eyes and imagine you are lying outside on a soft blanket, looking up at the night sky. The stars are twinkling above you, bright and beautiful. As you lie there, take a deep breath in through your nose, and breathe out slowly through your mouth. Imagine the stars twinkling every time you breathe in and out. Now, imagine that one of the stars is shining just for you. It's your special star. Every time you breathe in, feel its light filling your body with warmth and calm. As you breathe out, imagine your body getting more relaxed, sinking deeper into the soft blanket. Keep breathing slowly, and let your whole body feel relaxed and safe. When you're ready, slowly open your eyes, keeping that peaceful feeling as you drift into sleep."

4. Cloud Journey (5 minutes)

This meditation encourages relaxation and visualization, perfect for winding down.

Script:

"Close your eyes and take a deep breath in, then slowly breathe out. Now, imagine that you are floating on a soft, fluffy cloud in the sky. What color is your cloud? As you lie on the cloud, you feel completely safe and relaxed. The cloud is carrying you gently through the sky, and you can feel the soft breeze on your face. You're floating past trees, mountains, and rivers. You feel light and peaceful as your cloud moves slowly through the sky. Take a deep breath in, and as you breathe out, let your body relax even more. When you're ready, imagine your cloud gently lowering you back to the ground. Take a few more breaths, and when you feel ready, slowly open your eyes, bringing that peaceful feeling with you."

Tips for Creating a Meditation Routine with Kids

- **Start with a Regular Time:** Try meditating at the same time each day to make it part of the routine. Bedtime is a great time to practice relaxation meditations.
- **Use Positive Reinforcement:** Praise your child for trying meditation, even if they are fidgety or distracted. Building the habit is more important than getting it perfect.

- **Be Flexible:** Some days your child may not want to meditate, and that's okay. The goal is to create a positive experience, not to force them into it.

Meditating with your kids can help them develop lifelong tools for managing stress, building emotional resilience, and staying calm in difficult situations. By making mindfulness part of your family's routine, you're helping to foster a peaceful and connected home environment.

The Role of Prayer and Spirituality in Raising Well-Balanced Kids

Spirituality and practices like prayer can provide a foundation for emotional resilience and well-being. For many families, integrating these practices into daily life helps create a sense of purpose, inner peace, and connection that benefits both parents and children. Prayer and spirituality can instill a strong moral compass, teaching kids empathy, gratitude, and a sense of community.

Benefits of Spirituality and Prayer for Children

- **Emotional Resilience**: Regular prayer or meditation can help children manage stress and anxiety, fostering emotional stability.
- **Connection and Belonging**: Practicing spirituality as a family can strengthen bonds and reinforce a shared sense of values.
- **Mindfulness and Reflection**: Prayer and quiet moments encourage mindfulness, which can improve focus and self-regulation in children.

- **Gratitude and Positivity**: Regular gratitude practices tied to spirituality can enhance a child's outlook on life, promoting optimism and happiness.

How to Incorporate Prayer and Spiritual Practices

- **Daily Family Time**: Setting aside a few minutes for prayer, reflection, or gratitude sharing at the start or end of the day.
- **Affirmations and Intentions**: Helping children set positive intentions for their day can reinforce confidence and a sense of purpose.
- **Creating a Sacred Space**: Designating a cozy corner or space for prayer, meditation, or quiet time can make spirituality a more tangible part of your home.

Quick Energy Balancing Routine for Kids

This routine draws from energy practices like Reiki, Tai Chi, and Qi Gong, focusing on mindful movements, gentle touch, and breathwork. It helps ground and center children, promoting a sense of calm and balance in their bodies and minds.

Step 1: Grounding and Centering

- **Purpose**: Helps your child feel connected to the earth and grounded.
- **How to Do It**:

1. Have your child stand with their feet hip-width apart, arms relaxed at their sides.
2. Guide them to close their eyes and imagine roots growing from their feet into the earth, connecting them with the

ground.

3. Instruct them to take 3 deep breaths, inhaling through the nose and exhaling through the mouth. With each breath, they should imagine pulling up calming energy from the earth through their roots.

Step 2: Energy Sweep (Inspired by Reiki)

- **Purpose**: Clears negative energy and brings in calm.
- **How to Do It**:

1. Starting at the top of your child's head, gently place your hands a few inches above their body and move your hands down slowly toward their feet, imagining you are sweeping away any negative or unsettled energy.
2. Repeat this "energy sweep" 2-3 times, moving from the head down to the feet.
3. End by gently shaking your hands as if you are letting go of any excess energy.

Step 3: Tai Chi Flow – Holding the Ball

- **Purpose**: Promotes balance and a sense of control over emotions.
- **How to Do It**:

1. Have your child hold their hands out in front of them, as if they are cradling a ball of energy between their palms.
2. Instruct them to slowly move their hands in a circular motion, pretending to rotate the ball of energy. Encourage them to move slowly and smoothly.

3. After 1-2 minutes, have them switch the direction of the circle and continue for another minute.

Step 4: Qi Gong – Calming Breath with Hand Movements

- **Purpose**: Calms the nervous system and balances energy.
- **How to Do It**:

1. Have your child stand or sit comfortably with their hands resting in their lap or by their sides.
2. Instruct them to raise their arms up slowly, with palms facing the sky, as they take a deep breath in.
3. As they exhale, have them slowly lower their arms, turning the palms down, and imagine they are pushing out any tension or stress.
4. Repeat this movement 5 times, guiding them to breathe deeply and slowly.

Step 5: Heart Centering (Inspired by Reiki and Mindfulness)

- **Purpose**: Encourages emotional balance and a sense of calm.
- **How to Do It**:

1. Have your child place their hands over their heart, one on top of the other.
2. Instruct them to close their eyes and focus on their heartbeat.
3. Guide them to take 3 slow, deep breaths, imagining each breath filling their heart with warmth and peace.
4. Have them hold this position for 1-2 minutes, breathing

deeply and feeling the warmth from their hands.

This energy balancing routine helps calm and center children by engaging their breath, movement, and imagination. It can be done in just a few minutes and is a great tool for moments when kids feel anxious, overwhelmed, or restless.

Prioritizing emotional wellness equips children with the tools they need to handle life's challenges with resilience, confidence, and positivity. By teaching children to recognize and manage their emotions, practice mindfulness, and approach problems with a solution-oriented mindset, parents can foster emotional intelligence and resilience from a young age.

This chapter highlights the interconnectedness of the mind and body in holistic health. By focusing on emotional wellness, you ensure a well-rounded approach to raising emotionally strong and resilient children who are equipped to navigate life's challenges.

In the next chapter, we'll explore the transformative power of sleep and how it plays a crucial role in your child's growth and health. We'll dive into strategies for creating healthy sleep habits that support both emotional and physical well-being.

13

The Science of Sleep: Rest for Growth

Sleep is not merely a time for rest—it's an essential, regenerative process that fuels growth, brain development, and emotional stability, especially for children. The hours spent sleeping are some of the most crucial for your child's overall development. During sleep, their body repairs itself, consolidates learning, and processes emotions. A good night's sleep is a cornerstone of holistic health, helping children thrive physically, mentally, and emotionally.

Quality sleep is critical for physical growth, brain development, and emotional health. Ensuring your child gets enough rest is one of the most important aspects of their well-being. This chapter explores the science behind sleep, its impact on children's development, and practical strategies for creating a sleep-conducive environment that fosters healthy rest.

The Physiological Benefits of Sleep

Growth and Brain Development

Sleep is a crucial time when the body engages in essential processes that support overall health, growth, and development. It is far from a passive state; rather, it is an active period during which the body performs vital functions for repair, healing, and rejuvenation. This is particularly important for children, as they are in a continuous state of physical and mental growth.

1. **Physical Restoration** During sleep, the body works on repairing and building tissues. Growth hormone secretion, which peaks during deep sleep, stimulates tissue growth and muscle repair. This process is fundamental for children, as it supports their ongoing physical development. Additionally, the immune system becomes more active during sleep, producing cytokines that help fight infection and inflammation, thereby boosting overall immunity. Muscle recovery also occurs during sleep, allowing children to regain strength after daily activities and prepare for the next day.
2. **Brain Development and Cognitive Function** Sleep is essential for cognitive development, as it helps the brain process and consolidate information learned during the day. This process converts short-term memories into long-term storage, which is crucial for learning, language development, and overall cognitive growth in children. Another key process, known as synaptic pruning, occurs during sleep. This involves reducing excess neural connections to enhance the brain's efficiency and strengthen important pathways, supporting better cognitive functioning and emotional regulation.

Sleep also activates the glymphatic system, which clears waste products and toxins from the brain. This detoxification process is vital for maintaining neurological health and preventing cognitive decline. In children, these processes ensure that their developing brains function optimally, enhancing their learning abilities and emotional well-being.

3. Hormonal Regulation The regulation of hormones is another critical function that occurs during sleep. Growth hormone is released predominantly during deep sleep, aiding in cell regeneration, muscle and bone growth, and overall development in children. Melatonin, the hormone responsible for regulating the sleep-wake cycle, ensures that children can fall asleep and stay asleep, promoting restorative rest. Additionally, sleep helps lower cortisol levels, the stress hormone, allowing the body to recover from the day's stressors and reducing the risk of chronic stress, which can hinder growth and development.

4. Emotional and Mental Health Sleep plays a significant role in emotional processing and mental health. REM (rapid eye movement) sleep, associated with dreaming, helps children process emotions and manage stress. This contributes to improved emotional regulation and mental resilience. Sleep also aids in balancing neurotransmitters such as serotonin and dopamine, which regulate mood. Adequate sleep, therefore, leads to better mood stability and a positive outlook, essential for a child's emotional development.

5. Immune Support and Healing The body's healing processes are at their most active during sleep, making it essential for wound healing and recovery from illness. Proteins and enzymes that promote healing and fight infections function optimally during this time, which is why children recovering from injuries or illnesses need extra rest. Sleep also helps restore energy by replenishing glycogen stores, ensuring children have the stamina for play, learning, and exploration.

6. Growth and Development Sleep is vital for bone growth, especially during growth spurts when growth plates are more active. Cellular growth and division, essential for physical development and overall body maintenance, also occur at higher rates during sleep. This continuous cycle of growth and repair highlights why sufficient sleep is so crucial for children.

Sleep supports numerous restorative and developmental processes essential for children's health. From physical growth and immune function to brain development and emotional well-being, sleep lays the foundation for a child's overall health and future potential. Ensuring that children get adequate, high-quality sleep helps them thrive physically and mentally, setting the stage for lifelong wellness.

The Consequences of Sleep Deprivation

When children don't get enough sleep, the consequences are immediate and far-reaching. Sleep deprivation can lead to mood swings, irritability, and difficulty regulating emotions, making it harder for children to cope with stress. Over time, chronic sleep deprivation can also negatively affect behavior, concentration, and problem-solving skills, as well as contribute to long-term health issues like weakened immunity and childhood obesity.

A lack of sleep affects every aspect of a child's day-to-day life. From struggles with focus in the classroom to increased emotional outbursts, children who aren't well-rested are at a disadvantage. Understanding the critical role sleep plays in their health is the first step toward ensuring they get the rest they need.

Creating a Sleep-Conducive Environment

Optimizing the Bedroom for Rest

A calm, dark, and comfortable sleep environment is essential for promoting restful sleep. The bedroom should be free of distractions, such as electronics, bright lights, or loud noises, which can overstimulate children and make it harder for them to wind down. Instead, focus on creating a peaceful atmosphere with soft lighting, comfortable bedding, and soothing colors.

Some tips for optimizing the sleep environment include:

- **Darkness**: Consider using blackout curtains to eliminate light and create a calm setting that signals bedtime.
- **Cool Temperature**: A slightly cooler room helps the body relax and prepare for sleep.
- **Noise Control**: White noise machines or soft music can help mask disruptive sounds, while eliminating loud or sudden noises from the bedroom.

Healthy Bedtime Routines

Establishing a consistent bedtime routine helps signal to children that it's time to wind down and prepares their bodies for rest. A predictable sequence of calming activities before bed can make the transition from wakefulness to sleep easier. Some simple yet effective bedtime rituals include:

- **Bath Time**: A warm bath before bed helps relax the body and sets the stage for restful sleep.
- **Reading**: Reading a book together allows children to focus on calming activities and transition away from screen time.
- **Calming Music or White Noise**: Playing soft, calming music or white noise can create a peaceful environment and drown out any disruptive sounds.

By sticking to a routine, you help your child's body develop a natural rhythm that makes

Natural Sleep Remedies

Herbs and Supplements for Better Sleep

If your child has difficulty falling asleep or staying asleep, natural remedies can offer gentle and effective support without the need for medication. Here are some of the most child-safe and effective natural sleep aids:

Chamomile Tea: Chamomile is renowned for its calming properties. A warm cup of chamomile tea before bedtime can help relax the mind and body, making it easier for children to fall asleep and stay asleep.

Lavender Essential Oil: Lavender is well-known for its soothing aroma. A few drops of lavender essential oil on a pillow, in a diffuser, or added to a warm bath can create a calming environment that promotes relaxation and better sleep.

Magnesium: Magnesium helps relax muscles and improve overall sleep quality. Magnesium-rich foods like leafy greens, bananas, and pumpkin seeds can be included in your child's diet. Additionally, a warm bath with Epsom salts is a simple way to provide magnesium absorption through the skin.

Melatonin: Melatonin is a hormone naturally produced by the body to regulate sleep-wake cycles. For children who have trouble falling asleep, melatonin supplements can be a safe and effective option when used in low doses and under the guidance of a healthcare provider.

Valerian Root: Valerian root has mild sedative properties and can help calm a restless child. It can be given in small, age-appropriate doses as a tea or tincture to support sleep.

Lemon Balm: Lemon balm is a gentle herb that helps reduce nervousness and promotes calmness. It can be used as a tea or tincture to help children unwind before bedtime.

Passionflower: Known for its calming effects, passionflower can help children who have trouble falling asleep due to anxiety or restlessness. It can be taken as a tea or in tincture form in safe, appropriate doses.

Hops: Often used in combination with other calming herbs like chamomile and valerian, hops can help support relaxation and improve sleep quality. A mild hops tea or herbal blend can be used before bedtime.

Oat Straw: Oat straw is a nourishing herb that supports the nervous system and promotes relaxation. A warm oat straw tea or tincture can be given to children to help them feel calm and prepare for a restful night.

Ashwagandha: This adaptogenic herb can help balance cortisol levels and promote a sense of calm. It's safe for children in low doses and can be used as a tincture or added to warm milk before bedtime.

These gentle remedies support sleep naturally without the risk of side effects, making them safe options for children who may need a little extra help winding down at night. Always consult with a healthcare professional before introducing new supplements or herbs, especially for young children.

Addressing Sleep Issues Holistically

Common sleep disturbances, such as night terrors or difficulty falling asleep, can often be addressed through holistic strategies. For night terrors, ensuring that your child has a calm, consistent bedtime routine and a sleep-conducive environment can help. If your child has trouble falling asleep, consider introducing mindfulness exercises or relaxation techniques to help them relax their mind before bed.

Incorporating mindfulness into the bedtime routine, such as guided breathing exercises or a short meditation, can help children focus on the present moment and ease into sleep more easily.

The Impact of Earlier Bedtimes

One family shared their experience of making small but significant changes to their child's bedtime routine. After noticing that their son was becoming increasingly irritable and having trouble focusing at school, they decided to move his bedtime up by 30 minutes and remove all electronics from the bedroom. The result was almost immediate—he began waking up more refreshed, had fewer emotional outbursts, and his concentration improved in class. The simple shift to an earlier, more structured bedtime had a profound effect on his behavior and overall mood.

The Humorous Side of Bedtime Routines

Another family recounted a funny story about their attempt to implement a consistent bedtime routine. Initially, the children resisted the change, coming up with every excuse imaginable to delay bedtime—more water, another story, or needing a specific toy. However, after a few weeks of persistence, the routine took hold, and everyone in the household began to sleep better. The parents even noticed that they were benefitting from the routine, getting more rest themselves. What started as a struggle turned into a family-wide sleep improvement, proving that consistency pays off.

Adequate sleep is non-negotiable for a child's development. Sleep not only fuels physical growth but also supports emotional stability, cognitive function, and overall health. By prioritizing quality sleep, creating a conducive sleep environment, and establishing healthy bedtime routines, you're giving your child the foundation they need for long-term well-being.

This chapter emphasizes the importance of balance—just

as sleep is essential for physical growth, it is equally vital for emotional and cognitive wellness. Ensuring your child gets enough rest helps them grow stronger, both inside and out.

Next, we'll explore how holistic practices can help children develop resilience and cope with challenges, nurturing their inner strength and adaptability.

14

Navigating Challenges: Resilience Through Holistic Practices

Imagine facing a storm. Whether you get swept away or stand firm depends not just on your preparation, but on your resilience—your ability to adapt, bend without breaking, and grow stronger through adversity. Teaching children how to navigate life's inevitable challenges through holistic practices helps them develop this inner strength. By fostering resilience, you're giving them the tools to handle difficulties with grace, courage, and a mindset of growth.

Building resilience in children through holistic practices equips them to face life's challenges with confidence and adaptability. Holistic approaches, such as mindfulness, problem-solving, and community support, help children cultivate a growth mindset, allowing them to view setbacks as opportunities for learning rather than obstacles. This chapter explores how holistic practices foster resilience and prepare children for the challenges they will inevitably encounter.

Holistic Practices that Foster Resilience

Mind-Body Connection

Holistic practices that connect the mind and body—such as yoga, meditation, and mindfulness—are powerful tools for building resilience. These practices help children develop the ability to remain calm and centered during stressful situations, providing them with coping mechanisms they can rely on when faced with challenges.

- **Yoga** teaches children how to focus on their breath and movement, helping them develop both physical strength and mental clarity. Practicing yoga encourages self-awareness and emotional regulation, which are key components of resilience.
- **Meditation and Mindfulness** are equally important in teaching children how to stay grounded in the present moment. Mindfulness exercises can help children recognize their emotions without being overwhelmed by them, fostering emotional resilience. A simple practice like focusing on their breath during moments of anxiety can help children regain their calm and approach problems with a clear mind.

These practices create a strong foundation of self-regulation, enabling children to handle challenges with a calm and balanced approach, even in the face of uncertainty.

Sample Yoga Routine for Families

This gentle yoga routine is designed for parents and kids to practice together. It's perfect for fostering connection, relaxation, and developing strength and flexibility. The routine can be done in about 15–20 minutes.

1. Easy Pose (Sukhasana) with Deep Breathing (2–3 minutes)

- Sit cross-legged with your hands resting on your knees, palms up or down.
- Close your eyes and take slow, deep breaths. Inhale for a count of four, hold for a count of two, and exhale for a count of four.
- Encourage your child to focus on the rise and fall of their chest, promoting mindfulness and calm.

2. Cat-Cow Stretch (Marjaryasana-Bitilasana) (2 minutes)

- Come onto your hands and knees in a tabletop position.
- On an inhale, drop your belly, lift your tailbone and head for Cow Pose.
- On an exhale, round your back, tucking your chin to your chest for Cat Pose.
- Repeat slowly, syncing the movement with your breath.

3. Downward-Facing Dog (Adho Mukha Svanasana) (2 minutes)

- From tabletop, tuck your toes under and lift your hips up and back to form an inverted "V" shape.
- Press your palms firmly into the mat and lengthen your spine.
- Encourage your child to pretend they are a playful puppy stretching.

4. Cobra Pose (Bhujangasana) (1 minute)

- Lower yourself down to your belly and place your hands under your shoulders.
- Inhale and gently lift your chest while keeping your elbows slightly bent.
- Smile and look ahead, encouraging your child to imagine being a proud snake basking in the sun.

5. Child's Pose (Balasana) (2 minutes)

- Sit back on your heels and lower your torso forward, resting your forehead on the mat.
- Stretch your arms in front of you or rest them by your sides.
- This pose is calming and can be a great time for deep breathing.

6. Tree Pose (Vrksasana) (2 minutes)

- Stand up tall and find your balance on one foot.
- Place the sole of your other foot on your inner thigh or calf (avoid the knee).
- Bring your palms together at your heart or lift your arms overhead.
- Encourage your child to sway gently like a tree in the wind.

7. Seated Forward Bend (Paschimottanasana) (2 minutes)

- Sit with your legs stretched out in front of you.
- Reach forward, extending your arms toward your feet, and gently fold at your hips.

- Relax into the stretch and take deep breaths.

8. Happy Baby Pose (Ananda Balasana) (2 minutes)

- Lie on your back and bring your knees toward your chest.
- Hold the outsides of your feet with your hands and open your knees wider than your torso.
- Gently rock side to side, encouraging your child to giggle and imagine they are a playful baby.

9. Relaxation (Savasana) (3–5 minutes)

- Lie flat on your back with your arms by your sides and palms up.
- Close your eyes and focus on deep, slow breathing.
- Guide your child through a brief relaxation, asking them to imagine floating on a cloud or resting by a calm lake.

Closing Tip

End the session by sitting up in an easy pose and saying a short phrase together, such as "I am calm, I am strong, I am loved." This helps children leave the session with a sense of confidence and peace.

Yoga Routine for Holistic Wellness

Duration: 20–30 minutes

Purpose: To encourage relaxation, improve flexibility, and support mind-body balance.

1. Centering and Breathwork (3–5 minutes)

- **Easy Pose (Sukhasana):** Sit cross-legged on the floor, hands resting on your knees, palms facing up. Close your eyes and take deep, slow breaths in and out. Focus on the rise and fall of your abdomen. This helps calm the mind and set the tone for your practice.
- **Breathing Practice:** Practice deep diaphragmatic breathing or alternate nostril breathing (Nadi Shodhana) to further relax and center yourself.

2. Cat-Cow Stretch (Marjaryasana-Bitilasana) (2-3 minutes)

- **Instructions:** Come to an all-fours position with your hands directly under your shoulders and knees under your hips. Inhale as you drop your belly, lift your head, and arch your back (Cow Pose). Exhale as you round your spine, tucking your chin to your chest (Cat Pose). Repeat this motion with your breath, warming up the spine.

3. Downward-Facing Dog (Adho Mukha Svanasana) (2-3 minutes)

- **Instructions:** From all-fours, tuck your toes under and lift your hips toward the ceiling, creating an inverted V shape. Keep your knees slightly bent if needed and focus on lengthening your spine. Hold for a few deep breaths, then slowly lower back down to the mat.

4. Forward Fold (Uttanasana) (2-3 minutes)

- **Instructions:** Stand up tall and, on an exhale, hinge at the hips to fold forward, letting your head and arms dangle.

This helps release tension in the lower back and hamstrings. Bend your knees slightly if needed to avoid strain. Hold for several breaths before slowly rolling back up to a standing position.

5. Warrior II (Virabhadrasana II) (2 minutes each side)

- **Instructions:** Step your right foot forward and left foot back, turning your left foot slightly inward. Bend your right knee so it's over your ankle and extend your arms out parallel to the floor. Gaze over your right fingertips and hold for a few deep breaths. Switch sides and repeat.

6. Tree Pose (Vrksasana) (1-2 minutes each side)

- **Instructions:** Stand with feet hip-width apart. Shift your weight onto your left foot and place your right foot on your inner left thigh or calf (avoid the knee). Bring your hands to a prayer position at your chest or lift them overhead. Hold for a few breaths and switch sides. This pose helps improve balance and focus.

7. Seated Forward Bend (Paschimottanasana) (2-3 minutes)

- **Instructions:** Sit with your legs extended straight in front of you. Inhale to lengthen your spine and exhale as you fold forward, reaching for your feet or shins. Hold the stretch gently and breathe deeply, allowing the back of the body to relax.

8. Supine Twist (Supta Matsyendrasana) (1-2 minutes each

side)

- **Instructions:** Lie on your back and hug your knees to your chest. Drop both knees to the right as you extend your arms out in a T-shape and turn your head to the left. Hold the twist for a few breaths and switch sides. This pose helps release tension in the lower back and promotes spinal mobility.

9. Legs Up the Wall (Viparita Karani) (3-5 minutes)

- **Instructions:** Sit sideways next to a wall, then swing your legs up the wall as you lower your back onto the floor. Rest your arms by your sides and close your eyes. This gentle inversion promotes relaxation, reduces swelling in the legs, and calms the nervous system.

10. Final Relaxation (Savasana) (5 minutes)

- **Instructions:** Lie flat on your back with your arms relaxed at your sides and your legs extended. Close your eyes and take slow, deep breaths. Allow your body to fully relax and release any remaining tension. Stay in this pose for at least 5 minutes before gently coming back to a seated position.

End of Routine

Take a moment to express gratitude for your body and the time you've spent nurturing your well-being.

Meditation and Mindfulness Practices for Kids

Introducing meditation and mindfulness to children is a wonderful way to support their emotional well-being, enhance their focus, and develop self-regulation skills. These simple practices are designed to be engaging and accessible for children of all ages.

Why Meditation and Mindfulness Are Important for Kids

Children today face numerous stressors, from schoolwork to social interactions. Practicing mindfulness helps them develop the tools to manage emotions, stay calm under pressure, and build resilience. By incorporating fun and imaginative techniques, meditation can be both effective and enjoyable.

1. "Cookie Breathing" Exercise

This technique is a playful way to introduce deep breathing to young children and help them calm their minds.

How to Practice:

- Have your child sit comfortably or lie down with their hands on their belly.
- Ask them to imagine they are holding a warm, freshly baked cookie. Encourage them to inhale deeply through their nose as if they're smelling the delicious cookie.
- Hold the breath for a moment and then exhale slowly through their mouth, pretending to cool the cookie.
- Repeat for 5–10 rounds of breath, focusing on the rise and fall of their belly.

2. "Five Senses Check-In"

This practice helps kids become more aware of their surroundings and bring themselves into the present moment.

How to Practice:

- Guide your child to find a quiet spot to sit comfortably.
- Ask them to identify:
- **5 things they can see** (e.g., toys, pictures on the wall)
- **4 things they can touch** (e.g., soft blanket, their own clothing)
- **3 things they can hear** (e.g., birds chirping, distant traffic)
- **2 things they can smell** (e.g., a scented candle, fresh air)
- **1 thing they can taste** (e.g., a sip of water or a piece of fruit)
- This simple check-in helps children ground themselves, enhancing their sense of awareness and calm.

3. "Mindful Jar" Exercise

This activity is both visual and interactive, making it great for teaching mindfulness to young children.

Materials Needed:

- A clear jar or water bottle
- Water
- Glitter or small beads

How to Practice:

- Fill the jar with water and add glitter or small beads. Seal the lid tightly.

- Shake the jar and explain that the swirling glitter represents their thoughts when they're upset, excited, or anxious.
- Place the jar on a flat surface and watch the glitter slowly settle. As it settles, encourage your child to take deep, slow breaths and imagine their thoughts settling down, too.
- Discuss how, just like the glitter, their minds can become calmer with a moment of pause and breathing.

4. "Body Scan for Kids"

A body scan helps children become more aware of physical sensations and release tension.

How to Practice:

- Ask your child to lie down or sit comfortably and close their eyes.
- Begin by guiding their attention to their feet, asking them to notice any sensations or how their feet feel against the floor.
- Gradually move up through the legs, belly, chest, arms, and head, encouraging them to relax each area as they go.
- Finish with a few deep breaths, allowing them to feel completely relaxed.

5. "Cloud Watching Meditation"

Perfect for outdoor mindfulness, this exercise encourages observation and creative thinking.

How to Practice:

- Find a comfortable spot outside where you and your child

can lie on the grass or sit together.

- Ask your child to look at the clouds and watch their movement. Encourage them to imagine what the clouds might look like—animals, shapes, or scenes.
- While observing, practice slow, deep breathing and talk about how the clouds float by, similar to how thoughts come and go in our minds.

Tips for Parents:

- **Keep it Short and Fun:** Start with just a few minutes and gradually increase the time as your child becomes more comfortable with the practice.
- **Be Patient:** Mindfulness is a skill that takes practice. If your child becomes distracted, gently guide them back without judgment.
- **Make it a Routine:** Incorporating mindfulness into your daily schedule, such as before bed or after school, helps build consistency.

Benefits of Meditation and Mindfulness for Kids:

- Improves focus and concentration
- Reduces stress and anxiety
- Enhances emotional regulation
- Promotes better sleep
- Boosts overall well-being

Practicing these mindfulness exercises as a family can create moments of connection and calm, supporting both parents and children in their daily lives.

Empowering Problem-Solving and Adaptability

Resilience also comes from the ability to face challenges head-on and learn from setbacks. Encouraging children to tackle problems, rather than avoid them, fosters adaptability and a growth mindset. When children are empowered to find solutions to their problems, they become more confident in their ability to overcome difficulties.

Parents can nurture this by allowing their children to experience minor disappointments or challenges and guiding them through the process of problem-solving. Whether it's figuring out how to complete a difficult puzzle or handling a disagreement with a friend, these experiences teach children to approach challenges as opportunities for growth. By helping them break down problems into manageable steps, parents can reinforce the idea that no problem is insurmountable, and that failure is simply a step toward success.

Lessons from Adversity

Building Emotional and Physical Strength

Resilience is often built through overcoming small challenges, which strengthen both emotional and physical capabilities. Whether it's learning a new skill, coping with a minor failure, or dealing with disappointment, these experiences allow children to develop perseverance and emotional strength. When children learn that they can handle small setbacks, they become better equipped to face larger challenges later in life.

Encouraging your child to try new activities, even if they are difficult, helps build their confidence and resilience. For example, a child learning to ride a bike may fall several times before mastering the skill. Each fall provides a lesson in perseverance, and eventually, the child realizes that their determination leads to success. This kind of resilience builds emotional fortitude, helping children understand that challenges are temporary and surmountable.

Exercises and Activities to Build Resilience in Kids

Learning through adversity can help children develop crucial life skills, such as problem-solving, adaptability, and inner strength. Engaging in activities that promote mental, emotional, and physical strength allows kids to face challenges with confidence and grow into resilient individuals. Below are exercises and puzzles that can be integrated into daily routines to support holistic development.

1. Gratitude Journal

Purpose: Builds emotional strength by fostering a positive mindset.

How to Practice:

- Encourage your child to write down three things they're grateful for each day. These can be as simple as "playing with a friend" or "a sunny day."
- Reflecting on what they appreciate helps them focus on the good, even during tough times.

2. Mindful Movement and Balance Game

Purpose: Enhances physical coordination, mindfulness, and self-control.

How to Practice:

- Create a simple obstacle course using household items (pillows, cones, or books). Include challenges such as balancing on one foot or hopping on one leg.

- As they navigate the course, guide them to move slowly and breathe deeply to stay balanced and calm.
- This exercise helps them stay focused under pressure, improving both their physical and mental resilience.

3. Emotion Identification Puzzle

Purpose: Strengthens emotional awareness and regulation.

How to Practice:

- Create a set of cards with different emotions (e.g., happy, sad, frustrated, excited) and scenarios that might trigger those feelings.
- Ask your child to match the emotion to a scenario or share a time when they felt that emotion and how they handled it.
- This activity encourages them to recognize and talk about their feelings, fostering emotional intelligence and problem-solving.

4. Progressive Muscle Relaxation (PMR)

Purpose: Teaches physical relaxation and mental focus, helping to release tension.

How to Practice:

- Guide your child through a series of muscle tensing and relaxing exercises, starting from their feet and working up to their head.
- For example, say, "Squeeze your toes as tightly as you can for five seconds, then release and feel the difference."

- PMR helps children become aware of physical stress and learn how to let it go, promoting both mental and physical relaxation.

5. "What Would You Do?" Problem-Solving Cards

Purpose: Develops critical thinking and decision-making skills.
How to Practice:

- Create cards with different scenarios that present challenges, such as "What would you do if a friend wasn't sharing?" or "How would you handle feeling nervous about a test?"
- Have your child think through their response and discuss possible outcomes.
- This exercise teaches kids to think ahead and prepares them to handle real-life situations with a problem-solving approach.

6. Visualization Exercise: The Safe Place

Purpose: Improves emotional strength and mental resilience by teaching self-soothing techniques.
How to Practice:

- Ask your child to close their eyes and imagine a place where they feel completely safe and happy, like a favorite park or a cozy room.
- Guide them to describe this place with as much detail as possible—what it looks like, smells like, and how it makes them feel.

- Practicing this visualization can help children return to their "safe place" in their mind when facing anxiety or stress, giving them a tool for self-calming.

7. Puzzle Time: Brain Teasers and Riddles

Purpose: Builds mental strength, enhances problem-solving skills, and improves focus.
How to Practice:

- Set aside time each week for puzzles such as crosswords, sudoku, or age-appropriate brainteasers. You can even use simple riddles and ask your child to come up with answers.
- These activities challenge their thinking and help them learn to approach problems from different angles, strengthening cognitive flexibility.

8. Role-Playing Game

Purpose: Promotes social skills, empathy, and creativity.
How to Practice:

- Act out different scenarios with your child, like "meeting a new friend" or "asking for help when they're struggling."
- Role-playing helps children practice how to respond to various situations, build communication skills, and understand other people's perspectives.

9. Physical Strength Challenges

Purpose: Enhances physical resilience and confidence.
How to Practice:

- Introduce fun, simple physical challenges such as timed plank holds, wall sits, or animal walks (e.g., crab walks, bear crawls).
- Make it a game by timing them and celebrating their progress over time.
- These challenges help build strength and endurance, contributing to their physical well-being.

10. Affirmation Craft Time

Purpose: Boosts self-esteem and emotional resilience.
How to Practice:

- Help your child create a set of affirmation cards with positive phrases like "I am brave," "I am kind," or "I can handle tough situations."
- Encourage them to pick a card each day and repeat the phrase aloud.
- Positive affirmations can reframe negative thoughts and promote a resilient mindset.

Community Support in Times of Difficulty

Resilience is not built in isolation. A strong support network—family, friends, teachers, and community—plays a vital role in helping children bounce back from adversity. Knowing that they have a safety net of caring individuals gives children the confidence to take risks and face challenges, knowing they won't have to do it alone.

In times of difficulty, community support can provide emotional comfort, practical assistance, and guidance. Whether it's navigating a family crisis, struggling with school stress, or dealing with social challenges, children who feel supported by a loving community are more likely to recover quickly and emerge stronger. The presence of mentors, extended family, and peers reinforces the message that they are not alone in their struggles, which is essential for developing resilience.

Community Support: Holistic Ways to Help Your Child Through Difficult Times

Supporting children when they face difficulties requires a mindful and compassionate approach. Parents can play a pivotal role in helping their kids build resilience and emotional strength by using holistic, healthy strategies. Here are some effective ways to support your child:

1. Create a Safe Space for Open Communication

- **Encourage Open Dialogue:** Make it clear to your child that it's okay to talk about their feelings. Use phrases like, "I'm here to listen, not to judge," to foster an environment where they feel safe expressing themselves.
- **Active Listening:** Pay full attention when your child speaks. Validate their feelings by saying, "I understand that must be hard for you," to show empathy.

2. Practice Mindful Breathing Together

- **Guided Breathing Exercises:** Use simple exercises like "cookie breathing" or "balloon breathing" to help your child regulate emotions and reduce stress.
- **Calm Corner:** Create a quiet space at home with soft pillows, calming colors, and sensory toys where your child can go to practice mindfulness or take a break when they feel overwhelmed.

3. Use Gentle Physical Touch

- **Hugs and Massage:** Physical touch like a warm hug or a gentle back massage can have calming effects and help children feel secure and supported.
- **Hand-Holding or Lap Time:** For younger children, holding hands or sitting on a parent's lap can provide comfort and reassurance.

4. Integrate Art and Creativity

- **Art Therapy:** Encourage your child to express their emotions through drawing, painting, or crafting. Art is a powerful, non-verbal way for kids to process feelings.
- **Journaling Together:** Help older children start a journal where they can write down thoughts, emotions, or positive affirmations. Younger kids can draw pictures of their day or their feelings.

5. Incorporate Nature Time

- **Walks in Nature:** Spending time outside can greatly reduce stress and improve mood. Take your child for a walk, go to a park, or play in the yard to help them reconnect with nature.
- **Gardening Together:** Working on a small garden or planting flowers can teach patience and provide a calming, hands-on activity.

6. Practice Simple Yoga and Movement

- **Family Yoga Routine:** Do gentle yoga poses together to help release tension and build connection.
- **Dance Breaks:** A spontaneous dance session can lift spirits and release pent-up energy, creating a fun, shared experience.

7. Ensure Balanced Nutrition

- **Whole Foods:** Make sure your child is eating nutrient-rich foods, including fruits, vegetables, whole grains, and lean proteins. A healthy diet supports brain function and mood regulation.
- **Herbal Teas:** Age-appropriate, calming teas like chamomile (for older children) can help soothe anxiety and promote restful sleep.

8. Read Together

- **Books for Coping:** Choose books that focus on themes of overcoming challenges and building resilience. Stories can help children feel understood and inspired.

9. Model Healthy Coping Skills

- **Be the Example:** Show your child how you manage stress in healthy ways, such as through deep breathing, positive self-talk, or seeking support when needed.
- **Family Affirmation Time:** Create a daily or weekly ritual where everyone in the family shares positive affirmations or gratitude statements.

List of Resources for Holistic Support

- **Books for Kids and Parents:**
- *"The Whole-Brain Child" by Daniel J. Siegel and Tina Payne Bryson* – Provides strategies for fostering healthy emotional and mental development.
- *"Sitting Still Like a Frog" by Eline Snel* – A mindfulness book for kids and parents with guided exercises.
- *"Breathe Like a Bear" by Kira Willey* – Offers breathing and mindfulness exercises for young children.
- **Apps for Mindfulness:**
- *Headspace for Kids* – Engaging guided meditations tailored for different age groups.
- *Calm* – Has kid-friendly content that includes bedtime stories and meditation.
- *Smiling Mind* – Free mindfulness app with programs de-

signed for children.

- **Online Communities and Programs:**
- *Big Life Journal* – Offers resources that promote growth mindset and resilience in kids.
- *Child Mind Institute* – Provides articles and tools for supporting children's mental health.
- *GoZen!* – Online programs focused on emotional resilience and anxiety relief for kids.
- **Holistic Health Practices:**
- *Local Yoga Studios* – Many yoga studios offer kid-friendly or family classes.
- *Art Therapy Centers* – Consider looking for local or online art therapy workshops.
- *Holistic Health Practitioners* – Reach out to professionals who specialize in child-focused mindfulness, meditation, or nutritional support.

By integrating these strategies and utilizing these resources, parents can better support their children holistically through times of adversity, ensuring they grow with strength, resilience, and a sense of security.

A Family's Journey Through a Health Crisis

The Anderson family faced a major health crisis when their youngest child was diagnosed with a chronic illness. Initially overwhelmed by the diagnosis, the family turned to holistic strategies to find balance and recovery. They incorporated mindfulness exercises into their daily routine, practiced yoga as a family, and used herbal remedies to support their child's health. These practices helped them stay grounded and focused on healing, even during the most challenging moments. The family's commitment to holistic practices allowed them to navigate the emotional and physical challenges of the illness with resilience, ultimately emerging stronger as a unit.

A Child's Resilience Shining Through Tough Times

Samantha, an 8-year-old girl, had always been shy and nervous in new situations. When her family moved to a new city, she found the transition difficult, feeling isolated and overwhelmed by the unfamiliar environment. With her parents' guidance, she began using mindfulness exercises to calm her anxiety and yoga to stay centered. Over time, Samantha's natural resilience began to shine through. She made new friends, adapted to her new school, and learned to cope with the change using the holistic tools she had practiced at home. Samantha's story is a testament to how holistic coping tools can help children navigate tough times with emotional strength and adaptability.

Holistic practices foster resilience in children, equipping them with the emotional and mental tools to face challenges with confidence. By teaching children how to stay calm through mindfulness, encouraging problem-solving, and building a supportive community around them, parents can help children develop the strength and adaptability needed to thrive in the face of life's inevitable challenges.

Resilience is an essential element of balance and natural growth. By incorporating holistic practices into your child's life, you empower them to face difficulties with courage and confidence, ensuring they grow into emotionally strong and adaptable individuals.

In the following chapter, we'll discuss how to create a sustainable wellness blueprint for your family, incorporating holistic principles into your daily life to ensure long-term health and balance.

15

The Blueprint for Sustainable Wellness

Imagine crafting a blueprint for your dream home—carefully planned, personalized to your family's needs, and designed to stand the test of time. In the same way, building a sustainable wellness plan ensures long-term health and balance for your children and family. This blueprint is more than a collection of healthy habits; it's a thoughtful, comprehensive approach to wellness that integrates diet, lifestyle choices, and community involvement. Just as a well-designed home provides security and comfort, a well-crafted wellness plan provides the foundation for a lifetime of health and vitality.

A sustainable wellness blueprint incorporates diet, lifestyle, and community involvement to ensure that holistic health practices can be maintained for years to come. By designing a personalized wellness plan that meets your family's unique needs, you create a framework for lasting health and well-being. This chapter explores how to develop and implement a dynamic wellness plan that supports long-term growth and balance.

Developing a Family Wellness Plan

Personalizing Your Wellness Blueprint

Every family is different, and a one-size-fits-all approach to wellness rarely works. Personalizing your family's wellness plan involves tailoring health practices to your family's specific needs, goals, and challenges. Consider factors such as dietary preferences, existing health conditions, daily routines, and the unique needs of each family member. For some families, focusing on whole foods and meal planning may be the priority, while others might need to concentrate on improving sleep patterns or incorporating more mindfulness practices into their day.

Taking a personalized approach ensures that the wellness plan is practical, attainable, and suited to your family's lifestyle. The goal is to create a plan that can be realistically maintained and adjusted over time, as your family's needs evolve.

The Three Pillars of Holistic Wellness

A sustainable wellness plan is built on three key pillars: diet, lifestyle, and community. Each of these components plays a crucial role in promoting long-term health.

- **Diet**: The foods we eat are the foundation of health. A nutrient-dense, whole-foods diet provides the body with the vitamins, minerals, and energy needed to thrive. Incorporating herbal remedies and supplements when necessary helps fill any nutritional gaps and supports ongoing health.
- **Lifestyle**: Daily lifestyle choices, such as physical activity, mindfulness practices, and sleep routines, greatly impact overall wellness. Creating habits that support physical, mental, and emotional health is essential for maintaining balance and vitality.
- **Community**: A strong support system reinforces healthy habits and encourages collective wellness. Engaging with a

community that shares your holistic health values, whether through local groups, online forums, or wellness events, helps keep you accountable and provides valuable resources.

By focusing on these three pillars, families can create a wellness blueprint that is both dynamic and sustainable, providing a strong foundation for long-term health.

Implementing Holistic Practices

Diet as the Foundation

The foods we consume are the building blocks of wellness. By emphasizing whole foods, families can ensure that their bodies are receiving the nutrients they need for energy, growth, and immune function. A balanced diet rich in fruits, vegetables, lean proteins, whole grains, and healthy fats supports overall health and helps prevent chronic illness.

In addition to a whole-foods-based diet, herbal remedies and supplements can be incorporated to address specific health concerns or deficiencies. For example, a daily probiotic may support digestive health, while vitamin D supplements can boost immune function during winter months.

Meal planning and mindful eating are also essential parts of a sustainable wellness plan. By prioritizing home-cooked meals made from fresh, whole ingredients, families can create healthier eating habits that promote lifelong wellness.

Lifestyle Choices

Lifestyle is the second pillar of a sustainable wellness plan. Physical activity, whether it's family walks, yoga, or recreational sports, should be a regular part of your routine. Exercise not only improves physical health but also boosts mental clarity and emotional well-being.

Incorporating mindfulness practices, such as meditation or

breathing exercises, helps reduce stress and promotes mental and emotional balance. Teaching children mindfulness techniques from a young age equips them with valuable tools for managing their emotions and staying present.

Healthy sleep habits are another critical aspect of wellness. Establishing consistent bedtime routines and creating a sleep-conducive environment ensures that children get the rest they need for optimal growth and development. Prioritizing sleep helps the entire family stay energized, focused, and emotionally balanced.

Community Involvement

The final pillar of a sustainable wellness plan is community. Building a strong support network helps reinforce healthy habits and provides encouragement during challenging times. Joining local wellness groups, attending holistic health events, or participating in organic food co-ops are all ways to stay connected with others who share your values.

Community involvement is especially important for children, as it teaches them the importance of collective well-being. Engaging with a like-minded community can inspire positive lifestyle changes, provide resources for natural health practices, and strengthen your family's commitment to wellness.

A Family's Journey in Crafting Their Wellness Blueprint

The Carter family decided to overhaul their lifestyle after their youngest child developed recurring respiratory issues. They worked with a holistic health practitioner to develop a wellness blueprint tailored to their needs. They shifted to a whole-foods diet, removing processed foods and introducing supplements like vitamin C and zinc. They also began practicing yoga as a family, established consistent sleep routines, and joined a local wellness group focused on natural health. Over time, they saw significant improvements in their child's health, and the entire family felt more energetic and connected. The Carters continue to adjust their wellness plan as their needs evolve, ensuring it remains sustainable and effective.

Community Efforts for Health-Conscious Living

In a small town in Colorado, a group of families formed an organic food co-op to ensure access to fresh, local produce. The co-op not only provided affordable organic food but also fostered a sense of community around health-conscious living. Members of the co-op shared meal plans, gardening tips, and holistic health resources. Over time, the co-op expanded to include wellness workshops, mindfulness sessions, and herbal remedy exchanges. This collective action helped the community stay informed and committed to a lifestyle that prioritized health and sustainability.

Creating a sustainable wellness plan allows families to maintain balance and holistic health with long-term benefits for both parents and children. By focusing on diet, lifestyle, and community, families can build a wellness blueprint that supports ongoing health and fosters a positive, balanced approach to life.

This chapter reflects on the comprehensive approach to wellness, integrating diet, lifestyle, and community into a practical, sustainable blueprint. The wellness plan is dynamic, evolving with your family's needs, and serves as a guide for maintaining long-term health.

Next, we'll dive into the practical steps needed to integrate holistic principles into your daily routine, making these wellness practices a natural part of life.

Family Wellness Blueprint Worksheet

Step 1: Personalizing Your Family Wellness Plan

Reflection

Before developing your wellness blueprint, take a moment to reflect on your family's current health practices. Consider areas where you are already thriving and areas where you'd like to see improvement.

1. What are your family's current health strengths? (e.g., regular exercise, healthy meals, good sleep habits)

-
-
-
-

1. What are the areas where your family could improve? (e.g., more time outside, less screen time, more balanced meals)

-
-
-
-

1. Are there any specific health concerns or goals for your family? (e.g., better sleep, improved digestion, stress management)

-
-
-
-

Step 2: The Three Pillars of Wellness

Use the following sections to build your personalized wellness blueprint, focusing on **diet**, **lifestyle**, and **community involvement**.

1. Diet: Building Healthy Habits

Current Diet Assessment

How would you describe your family's current eating habits?

- What are the go-to meals and snacks for your family?
-
-
- How often do you cook meals at home versus eating out or ordering in?
-
-

Goal Setting

What changes would you like to make in your family's diet to support better health?

- Introduce more whole foods (e.g., fruits, vegetables, whole grains):
-
-

- Limit processed or sugary foods:
-
-
- Include supplements or herbal remedies:
-
-

Action Plan

List three specific actions you can take to improve your family's diet:

1.
2.
3.
4.
5.
6.

2. Lifestyle: Daily Routines for Wellbeing

Current Lifestyle Assessment

Reflect on your family's daily routines:

- How much physical activity does your family get each week? (e.g., walks, sports, playtime)
-
-
- Do you practice mindfulness or relaxation techniques as a family?
-
-

- How consistent are your family's sleep routines?
-
-

Goal Setting

What lifestyle changes would support your family's physical and emotional health?

- Increase physical activity (e.g., family walks, yoga, sports):
-
-
- Incorporate mindfulness or meditation practices:
-
-
- Improve bedtime routines for better sleep:
-
-

Action Plan

List three specific actions you can take to improve your family's lifestyle:

1.
2.
3.
4.
5.
6.

3. Community Involvement: Building Support Networks

Current Community Assessment

How involved is your family in wellness-focused communities or activities?

- Do you have a support network of like-minded individuals for health and wellness advice?
-
-
- How often do you participate in community wellness events or activities?
-
-

Goal Setting

What steps can you take to strengthen your family's connection to a health-conscious community?

- Join or create a local organic food co-op or wellness group:
-
-
- Participate in community activities that promote health and wellness:
-
-
- Seek support from holistic health practitioners or groups:
-
-

Action Plan

List three specific actions you can take to get more involved in your wellness community:

1.
2.
3.
4.
5.
6.

Step 3: Putting It All Together – Your Family Wellness Blueprint

Now that you've set goals and identified areas for improvement, outline your family's **Wellness Blueprint** below. Be sure to include actionable steps in **diet**, **lifestyle**, and **community involvement**.

Diet Goals:

-
-
-
-

Lifestyle Goals:

-
-
-
-

Community Involvement Goals:

-
-
-
-

Next Steps:

What are the first steps you will take to implement this wellness plan in your daily life?

-
-
-
-

Step 4: Review and Adjust Over Time

Wellness is a dynamic journey, and your family's needs may change over time. Schedule regular check-ins (e.g., monthly or quarterly) to review your family's wellness blueprint and make adjustments as needed.

- **Next Review Date:** ______________________________________ ____________________

16

Practical Steps: Applying Holistic Principles Daily

Picture yourself intentionally crafting each day with purpose and a vision for health. Just as an artist adds strokes to a canvas, small, consistent actions shape your family's well-being. The secret to maintaining holistic wellness lies not in grand gestures but in the small, practical steps you take every day. These daily habits, woven into the rhythm of your life, create a sustainable foundation for long-term health.

Small, consistent actions are key to applying and maintaining holistic health principles in daily life. By integrating these practices into your daily routine, holistic wellness becomes a natural part of your family's lifestyle—an achievable, sustainable journey that benefits everyone.

Integrating Holistic Practices into Daily Life

Morning and Evening Routines

The way we start and end our days sets the tone for everything in between. Simple, mindful routines can make a significant difference in the overall well-being of your family.

- **Morning Practices**: Begin the day with intention. Incorporate meditation or a few minutes of stretching to ground yourself before the busyness begins. A nutritious breakfast, rich in whole foods like fruits, grains, and proteins, ensures that everyone starts the day nourished and energized. Something as simple as adding chia seeds to smoothies or having herbal teas in the morning can subtly reinforce healthy habits.
- **Evening Wind-Down**: Bedtime routines matter as much as mornings. Unplug from screens an hour before bed, opting instead for a calming ritual such as reading, light stretching, or guided breathing exercises. Small actions like using lavender essential oil in a diffuser or drinking a warm cup of chamomile tea can help relax the body and mind for restful sleep.

Daily Nutritional Habits

Food is a central pillar of holistic wellness, but it doesn't have to feel overwhelming. Incorporating whole foods, herbs, and supplements into your meals and snacks can be simple and efficient, even on the busiest days.

- **Balanced Meals**: Focus on whole foods that are easy to prepare and packed with nutrients. For example, prepare grain bowls with quinoa, vegetables, and lean proteins that can be assembled quickly. Smoothies are another quick and nutritious option, where you can add greens, seeds, or herbal powders for an extra health boost.
- **Herbs and Supplements**: Integrating herbal remedies like elderberry syrup for immunity or magnesium for better sleep can become part of your daily routine. Supplements

like probiotics or multivitamins can be added to meals to support overall health without disrupting your schedule.

The key is to build habits that fit naturally into your family's life making one small change at a time, rather than overwhelming your routine with drastic changes.

Holistic Dental Health: Natural Approaches to Oral Care

Dental health is a natural part of most healthy morning and evening routines. It is a critical part of overall wellness, and a holistic approach to oral care can help prevent cavities, gum disease, and other common issues while supporting the body's natural healing processes. By focusing on nutrition, digestion, and natural oral care products, you can promote strong, healthy teeth and gums without relying solely on conventional products.

1. **Nourishing Your Teeth from Within**

Good dental health begins with proper nutrition, which strengthens teeth from the inside out. Your body requires specific vitamins and minerals to maintain strong enamel and healthy gums, and getting these through whole foods and supplements can reduce the risk of cavities and tooth decay.

- **Calcium and Bone Meal**: Calcium is essential for maintaining strong teeth and bones. One powerful way to support dental health is by adding **bone meal** to your diet. Bone meal, a powdered form of ground animal bones, is a rich source of calcium, phosphorus, and magnesium—all of which are vital for remineralizing teeth. You can add bone meal to smoothies, soups, or baked goods to boost your calcium intake. Be sure to choose high-quality, food-grade bone meal.

- **Vitamin D**: Vitamin D helps the body absorb calcium and phosphorus, which are critical for maintaining strong teeth. Getting plenty of sunlight and consuming foods like fatty fish, fortified dairy products, or egg yolks ensures you maintain adequate levels of vitamin D.
- **Magnesium**: Magnesium balances calcium in the body and supports the remineralization of teeth. Include magnesium-rich foods such as leafy greens, almonds, and pumpkin seeds in your diet, or consider supplementation.
- **Vitamin K2**: This vitamin works in tandem with calcium and vitamin D, directing calcium to the bones and teeth while preventing it from depositing in the arteries. Foods like grass-fed butter, fermented foods (such as sauerkraut), and organ meats are excellent sources of vitamin K2.

2. Proper Digestive Health and Cavity Prevention

Good digestion plays a vital role in dental health. If your digestive system isn't functioning optimally, your body may struggle to absorb the essential nutrients required to keep teeth strong and prevent cavities.

- **Gut Health and Nutrient Absorption**: Poor digestion can result in nutrient deficiencies, which directly impact tooth and gum health. Maintaining a healthy gut by consuming probiotics (found in yogurt, kefir, and fermented vegetables) and prebiotic-rich foods (such as garlic, onions, and asparagus) ensures that your body can efficiently absorb calcium, magnesium, and other vital nutrients.
- **Acid Reflux and Tooth Decay**: Acid reflux or indigestion can expose your teeth to stomach acid, which erodes enamel

and contributes to cavities. Managing reflux through a balanced diet, avoiding acidic foods (like sodas and citrus), and including alkaline foods (like leafy greens) can protect your teeth from unnecessary wear.

- **Saliva and Digestive Enzymes**: Saliva plays an important role in breaking down food and maintaining a healthy oral environment. Chewing thoroughly and incorporating digestive enzymes or natural chewing aids, like fennel seeds, can stimulate saliva production, which helps neutralize acids and wash away food particles that contribute to plaque buildup.

3. Natural Oral Care Products

Switching to natural oral care products can support your dental health while avoiding the chemicals found in conventional products.

- **Fluoride-Free Toothpaste**: Many holistic families prefer fluoride-free toothpaste. Look for toothpaste with natural ingredients like baking soda, coconut oil, or activated charcoal, which help clean teeth and fight bacteria without harsh additives.
- **Oil Pulling**: This ancient practice involves swishing a tablespoon of oil (such as coconut or sesame oil) in your mouth for 10-20 minutes. Oil pulling helps reduce harmful bacteria, freshens breath, and supports gum health. Regular oil pulling may also help reduce plaque and whiten teeth.
- **Bone Broth and Tooth Remineralization**: Consuming nutrient-dense bone broth regularly provides collagen, calcium, and magnesium, all of which support healthy teeth and gums. The minerals in bone broth contribute to the

remineralization of teeth, protecting against cavities.

4. Daily Habits for Dental Health

Daily habits play a significant role in maintaining oral health, especially when combined with holistic, natural practices.

- **Brush Twice a Day**: Use a soft-bristled toothbrush with a natural toothpaste to gently clean teeth, focusing on the gumline. Brushing in the morning and before bed removes plaque and reduces the risk of decay.
- **Floss Regularly**: Flossing is essential for removing food particles between teeth. Look for natural, biodegradable floss alternatives, like silk floss, to minimize environmental impact while promoting dental health.
- **Hydrate**: Drinking plenty of water throughout the day helps maintain saliva production and washes away harmful bacteria that can lead to tooth decay.
- **Chew Crunchy Vegetables**: Foods like celery, carrots, and apples act as natural toothbrushes, scrubbing away plaque and stimulating saliva production, which protects against cavities.

5. Holistic Solutions for Common Dental Issues

Holistic approaches can help address common dental concerns in natural ways.

- **Gum Health**: If you're dealing with gum irritation or inflammation, try rinsing with saltwater or applying clove oil, which has natural antibacterial and anti-inflammatory properties.
- **Tooth Sensitivity**: For sensitive teeth, use a natural desensi-

tizing toothpaste with ingredients like potassium nitrate or arginine. Additionally, ensure that you're getting adequate calcium, magnesium, and vitamin D for stronger enamel.

- **Cavity Prevention**: Incorporating more calcium-rich foods, bone meal, and digestive support into your diet, along with regular brushing and flossing, can help prevent cavities naturally. Remineralizing tooth powder (made with ingredients like calcium carbonate and clay) can be used to strengthen enamel and reduce the risk of decay.

Nourish and Protect Your Teeth with Natural Practices

Holistic dental health goes beyond brushing and flossing—it involves nourishing your body from the inside out and supporting proper digestion to maintain strong, healthy teeth. By incorporating bone meal, focusing on gut health, and using natural oral care products, you can protect your teeth from cavities and promote long-term oral wellness.

Overcoming Common Challenges

Dealing with Resistance to Change

Change can be hard, especially when introducing new habits to family members who might be resistant. Children may balk at unfamiliar foods, and adults may struggle to adjust to new routines.

- **Making It Fun**: Engage children by involving them in the process. Let them help pick ingredients for meals or choose fun ways to move their bodies through outdoor play or family yoga. Turn meal prep into a family activity, where children can learn about the nutritional benefits of the foods they're eating.

- **Gradual Changes**: Start small and gradually introduce changes. For example, swap sugary snacks for fruit smoothies or include a daily mindful moment before bedtime. By slowly incorporating new habits, your family is less likely to feel overwhelmed and more likely to embrace these healthy shifts.

Time Management

Finding time for holistic practices in a busy schedule can be challenging, but it's possible with planning and intention.

- **Meal Prepping**: Dedicate time during the weekend to plan and prepare meals for the week. Pre-cut vegetables, prepare smoothie ingredients in advance, and batch cook grains or soups that can be reheated easily. This simplifies weekday meals and ensures you always have healthy options on hand.
- **Short, Intentional Practices**: Mindfulness doesn't have to mean hours of meditation. A five-minute breathing exercise before bed or stretching while watching TV can easily fit into your day. Focus on integrating small actions that contribute to well-being without feeling like additional tasks.

Tools and Resources for Holistic Living

Holistic Health Resources

There are plenty of tools and resources available to support your holistic health journey. Consider incorporating these into your routine for ongoing education and inspiration:

- **Books**: Titles on holistic health, mindfulness, or herbal remedies can deepen your understanding of natural wellness. Look for family-friendly resources that offer practical advice.

- **Podcasts & Apps**: Podcasts on wellness topics or meditation apps (like Calm or Headspace) can provide accessible ways to practice mindfulness or learn new health tips.
- **Local Groups & Communities**: Joining local wellness groups, organic food co-ops, or attending holistic health workshops can help reinforce your family's commitment to natural health.

Adapting Holistic Practices Over Time

Holistic health is a dynamic process, and your family's needs will evolve over time. Be flexible in adjusting your routines as your children grow and life changes.

- **Seasonal Adjustments**: Adapt your family's diet, activities, and wellness practices to the seasons. For instance, in winter, focus on warming foods and herbs to boost immunity, while in summer, emphasize cooling foods and hydration.
- **Life Stage Changes**: As your children grow, their health needs will change. Be prepared to adjust their diet, sleep routines, and mindfulness practices to support them at each stage of development.

A Family's Transition to Daily Holistic Practices

The Martinez family wanted to integrate more holistic health practices into their daily life, but with busy work and school schedules, it felt overwhelming at first. They decided to start small by introducing herbal teas in the evening, swapping out processed snacks for homemade fruit smoothies, and adding five minutes of family meditation before bed. Over time, these small shifts made a significant impact. The children became more engaged in meal prep, the parents noticed they were less stressed, and everyone began sleeping better with the new bedtime routine. The gradual transition made it easy to maintain these habits without disrupting their busy schedules.

Humorous Account of Small Daily Changes

The Thompson family started their wellness journey by trying out yoga together. At first, the kids giggled through every pose, unable to focus, while the parents felt stiff and awkward. But after a few weeks of persistence, yoga became a fun family ritual. Even the family dog started joining in, curling up on the yoga mat during savasana. This small change—just 15 minutes a day—brought the family closer, and they found themselves laughing and enjoying the process, all while getting fitter and more relaxed.

Small, consistent, and intentional actions are the key to integrating holistic principles into daily life. By focusing on manageable changes, like incorporating healthy meals, short mindfulness practices, and creating consistent routines, holistic wellness becomes a natural and sustainable part of your family's lifestyle. Over time, these small shifts add up to long-term health and balance.

This chapter emphasizes the importance of daily choices in shaping a holistic lifestyle. By making wellness practices a natural part of your everyday routine, you create a foundation for sustainable, long-term health that benefits your entire family.

In the final chapter, we'll explore how embracing holistic health principles leads to lifelong wellness for both parents and children, creating a lasting legacy of health and balance.

17

Embracing Lifelong Holistic Health

Imagine a tree growing, its roots deepening and its branches reaching upward through the changing seasons. Just as a tree's growth is continuous, so too is health a lifelong journey, not a final destination. The holistic health practices we begin in childhood lay the foundation for wellness that extends into adolescence and adulthood. As your children grow, these practices will evolve with them, guiding them toward a life of balance, independence, and fulfillment.

The journey of raising well-balanced children is ongoing, requiring a lifelong commitment to holistic health beyond childhood. By instilling holistic principles early on, you provide your children with the tools they need to care for their own health, fostering independence, resilience, and long-term wellness. This chapter explores how holistic practices, started in childhood, extend into adulthood and become a lifelong path to health.

The Benefits of Lifelong Holistic Living

Health Benefits Beyond Childhood

The principles of holistic health that support your child's

growth and development don't end in childhood. As children move into adolescence and adulthood, these practices continue to offer profound benefits. Regular physical activity, mindful eating, stress management, and emotional balance are habits that help prevent chronic illnesses, enhance mental clarity, and support emotional resilience throughout life.

Holistic health teaches children to listen to their bodies, understand their needs, and make informed choices about their health. By growing up in an environment that emphasizes natural wellness, children are more likely to carry these values with them into adulthood, promoting long-term health and well-being.

Raising Health-Conscious Adults

One of the greatest gifts you can give your children is the ability to care for their own health. By involving them in holistic health practices from a young age—whether through teaching them how to cook nutritious meals, practice mindfulness, or understand the importance of sleep—you're preparing them to become independent, health-conscious adults.

As they grow older, children who have been raised with holistic principles are more likely to prioritize their physical and emotional well-being. They develop the confidence to make health-related decisions on their own, whether it's choosing whole foods, incorporating natural remedies, or managing stress in healthy ways. In turn, these practices promote a fulfilling and balanced lifestyle, one that they can carry into their own families in the future.

The Role of Essential Vitamins in Lifelong Development

Vitamins play a critical role in supporting physical and cognitive development, particularly during childhood and adolescence. As children grow, their nutritional needs change, and ensuring they receive the right vitamins at each stage is essential for lifelong health.

Infancy and Early Childhood (0-5 years)

During early development, children need specific vitamins to support rapid growth, brain development, and a strong immune system.

- **Vitamin D**: Vital for bone growth and the development of a healthy immune system.
- **Food Sources**: Fortified milk, fatty fish (such as salmon), and eggs. Vitamin D supplementation is often recommended for young children, especially in areas with limited sunlight.
- **Vitamin A**: Supports vision, immune health, and skin development.
- **Food Sources**: Carrots, sweet potatoes, spinach, and eggs.
- **Vitamin C**: Important for the growth and repair of tissues and helps the body absorb iron.
- **Food Sources**: Citrus fruits (oranges, lemons), strawberries, bell peppers, and broccoli.
- **Iron**: Supports brain development and is crucial for healthy red blood cells.
- **Food Sources**: Iron-fortified cereals, spinach, lentils, and lean red meat.

School-Age Children (6-12 years)

As children grow and their physical activity increases, so do their nutritional needs. Key vitamins at this stage are critical for energy, brain function, and immune health.

- **B Vitamins (B6, B12)**: Essential for energy production, brain health, and red blood cell formation.
- **Food Sources**: Whole grains, fish, chicken, beans, and eggs.
- **Calcium**: Vital for bone and teeth development, especially as children grow taller and stronger.
- **Food Sources**: Dairy products (milk, yogurt, cheese), leafy greens like kale, and fortified plant-based milks.
- **Zinc**: Supports immune health and cell growth, which is important as children begin puberty.
- **Food Sources**: Chickpeas, nuts, seeds, beef, and whole grains.
- **Magnesium**: Crucial for muscle and nerve function and helps regulate blood sugar.
- **Food Sources**: Leafy greens, nuts, seeds, avocados, and bananas.

Adolescence (13-18 years)

Adolescence is a period of rapid growth and hormonal changes, and it's crucial to ensure teens get the vitamins and nutrients they need to support these changes.

- **Vitamin E**: Acts as an antioxidant, supporting skin health and protecting cells from damage.
- **Food Sources**: Nuts, seeds, spinach, and sunflower oil.
- **Folate (Vitamin B9)**: Supports cell growth, especially important during periods of rapid growth and for girls reaching reproductive age.

- **Food Sources**: Leafy greens, beans, citrus fruits, and fortified cereals.
- **Omega-3 Fatty Acids**: Essential for brain health, especially during late adolescence, when the brain continues to develop.
- **Food Sources**: Fatty fish (salmon, mackerel), walnuts, flaxseeds, and chia seeds.
- **Vitamin K**: Supports blood clotting and bone health.
- **Food Sources**: Kale, spinach, broccoli, and green peas.

Adulthood and Ongoing Health

As your children grow into adulthood, maintaining their intake of essential vitamins is crucial for long-term health, including energy, skin health, immune function, and mental clarity.

- **Vitamin D**: Continues to be vital for bone health, especially for preventing osteoporosis later in life.
- **Food Sources**: Fatty fish, fortified foods, and sunlight exposure.
- **Vitamin B12**: Essential for nerve function and energy production.
- **Food Sources**: Meat, fish, dairy products, and fortified cereals.
- **Antioxidants (Vitamins A, C, E)**: Protect the body from oxidative stress and support healthy aging.
- **Food Sources**: Colorful fruits and vegetables (berries, oranges, leafy greens), nuts, and seeds.
- **Magnesium**: Helps maintain muscle and nerve function, regulates blood sugar, and supports overall wellness.
- **Food Sources**: Almonds, pumpkin seeds, dark chocolate,

and leafy greens.

Meal Plan 1: For School-Age Children (6-12 years)

Breakfast: Spinach & Cheese Scrambled Eggs (Vitamin A, Calcium, B Vitamins, Zinc)

- 2 eggs
- 1 cup fresh spinach
- ¼ cup shredded cheese (cheddar or mozzarella)
- Salt and pepper to taste
- 1 tsp olive oil

Snack: Apple Slices with Almond Butter (Vitamin C, Magnesium)

- 1 apple, sliced
- 2 tbsp almond butter

Lunch: Chicken Quinoa Salad (B Vitamins, Magnesium, Zinc, Iron)

- ½ cup cooked quinoa
- 3 oz cooked chicken breast, cubed
- ½ cup cucumber, diced
- ¼ cup cherry tomatoes, halved
- 1 tbsp olive oil
- 1 tsp lemon juice
- Salt and pepper to taste

Snack: Greek Yogurt with Berries and Chia Seeds (Calcium,

Vitamin D, Omega-3)

- ½ cup plain Greek yogurt
- ¼ cup mixed berries (blueberries, strawberries)
- 1 tsp chia seeds

Dinner: Salmon with Roasted Sweet Potatoes and Broccoli (Vitamin D, Omega-3, Vitamin A, Vitamin C)

- 1 salmon fillet (3-4 oz)
- 1 sweet potato, cubed
- 1 cup broccoli florets
- 1 tbsp olive oil
- Salt, pepper, and garlic powder to taste

Dessert: Homemade Fruit Smoothie (Magnesium, Vitamin C)

- 1 banana
- ½ cup frozen berries
- 1 tsp flaxseed
- 1 cup almond milk (fortified with calcium and vitamin D)

Meal Plan 2: For Adolescents (13-18 years)

Breakfast: Greek Yogurt Parfait (Calcium, Vitamin D, Vitamin C, Omega-3)

- ½ cup Greek yogurt
- ¼ cup granola (choose one low in added sugar)
- ¼ cup mixed berries (blueberries, raspberries)
- 1 tsp chia seeds or flaxseeds

Snack: Carrot Sticks with Hummus (Vitamin A, Magnesium)

- 1 large carrot, cut into sticks
- 2 tbsp hummus

Lunch: Turkey & Avocado Wrap (B Vitamins, Zinc, Magnesium, Vitamin E)

- 1 whole-grain wrap
- 3 oz sliced turkey breast
- ¼ avocado, sliced
- 1 slice of cheese (optional for extra calcium)
- Lettuce and tomato slices

Snack: Mixed Nuts & Seeds (Magnesium, Vitamin E)

- ¼ cup mixed nuts (almonds, walnuts, cashews)
- 1 tbsp sunflower or pumpkin seeds

Dinner: Lemon Garlic Chicken with Roasted Vegetables (Iron, Zinc, Vitamin C)

- 1 chicken breast (3-4 oz), marinated in lemon juice, garlic, and olive oil
- 1 cup broccoli florets
- 1 red bell pepper, sliced
- 1 tbsp olive oil
- Salt, pepper, and garlic powder to taste

Recipe:

1. Preheat oven to 400°F (200°C).
2. Marinate the chicken breast in lemon juice, garlic, olive oil, salt, and pepper. Set aside.
3. Toss broccoli and bell pepper in olive oil, salt, and garlic powder. Spread on a baking sheet.
4. Roast vegetables for 20 minutes. While they roast, grill or pan-sear the chicken breast until fully cooked, about 5-7 minutes per side, depending on thickness.
5. Serve chicken with roasted vegetables and a side of brown rice or quinoa.

Dessert: Dark Chocolate Almond Clusters (Magnesium, Antioxidants)

- 2 oz dark chocolate (70% cocoa or higher)
- 1/4 cup almonds

Recipe:

1. Melt dark chocolate in the microwave or over a double boiler.
2. Stir in almonds, then spoon the mixture onto a baking sheet lined with parchment paper. Let cool in the fridge until set.

Celebrating Milestones and Progress

Recognizing Holistic Growth

Holistic health is a journey, and it's important to celebrate the milestones along the way. Whether it's overcoming a specific health challenge, mastering a new skill like preparing nutritious meals, or cultivating mindfulness, these achievements deserve recognition. Celebrating these "small wins" not only reinforces healthy habits but also fosters a sense of accomplishment and motivation to continue the journey.

As a family, you can celebrate by recognizing the progress you've made together. This could be as simple as a family hike to mark a year of healthier living or preparing a favorite meal together as a reward for reaching a wellness goal. These celebrations create positive memories associated with health and reinforce the idea that wellness is something to be enjoyed, not a chore to be checked off.

Maintaining Balance Over Time

As your children grow, your family's holistic practices will need to evolve. Adolescents and young adults face different health challenges than younger children, and it's important to adapt your wellness routines to meet these changing needs. For example, as teenagers become more independent, they may need guidance on how to manage stress, maintain healthy relationships, and make mindful choices about food and physical activity on their own.

Continuing to provide support as they navigate these changes is key. Encourage them to explore new aspects of wellness—whether it's joining a yoga class, learning about herbal remedies, or creating their own healthy routines. By giving them the tools and confidence to care for their health, you help them maintain balance as they step into adulthood.

Personal Growth Through Holistic Practices

The Gomez family's journey into holistic health began with small changes: swapping out processed snacks for whole foods and incorporating daily meditation. Over time, these small shifts grew into a lifestyle, and the family noticed improvements in energy, mood, and overall health. As the children grew older, they took ownership of their health, learning to cook healthy meals and manage their emotions through mindfulness. What started as a family project became a lifelong practice, and the Gomez children now carry those principles into their own adult lives.

Children Embracing Holistic Health into Adulthood

One family shared how their daughter, Emily, who had grown up with a strong emphasis on natural wellness, continued to use holistic practices as she entered college. Despite the stress of university life, she maintained her yoga practice, prepared nutritious meals in her dorm, and used natural remedies to manage stress and stay balanced. Emily's ability to apply the holistic principles she learned in childhood to her adult life helped her stay grounded, healthy, and resilient through the challenges of college.

Holistic living is a lifelong path that leads to wellness, independence, and fulfillment. By instilling holistic health practices in your children from a young age, you not only support their growth and development but also provide them with the tools they need to lead healthy, balanced lives as adults. These practices create a foundation for long-term well-being that benefits both parents and children, fostering independence, resilience, and a deep connection to natural health.

This chapter highlights the long-term benefits of holistic health practices, emphasizing that the journey of wellness continues throughout life. The holistic principles you instill today set the stage for lifelong health and independence, creating a legacy of wellness that extends beyond childhood.

As you reach the end of this book, take a moment to reflect on the journey you've begun with your family. Embracing holistic health is not about perfection; it's about making intentional choices, one step at a time, that lead to a healthier, more balanced life. The principles and strategies shared throughout this book are here to guide you, but the real magic happens in the daily decisions you make for yourself and your family.

I encourage you to take the next steps in your personal and family health journey. Whether it's incorporating more whole foods into your diet, practicing mindfulness together, or connecting with your community, every action counts. As you continue on this path, remember that holistic health is a lifelong commitment—one that brings lasting benefits for both parents and children. Your journey to lifelong wellness starts today.

Appendix

100 Resources for Crunchy Moms

Books

1. "The Vaccine-Friendly Plan" by Paul Thomas, M.D.
2. "The Nourishing Traditions Book of Baby & Child Care" by Sally Fallon Morell
3. "Gentle Birth, Gentle Mothering" by Dr. Sarah Buckley
4. "The Whole-Brain Child" by Daniel J. Siegel and Tina Payne Bryson
5. "The Fourth Trimester" by Kimberly Ann Johnson
6. "The Womanly Art of Breastfeeding" by La Leche League International
7. "The Natural Baby" by Samantha Quinn
8. "No-Drama Discipline" by Daniel J. Siegel
9. "How to Raise a Healthy Child in Spite of Your Doctor" by Dr. Robert S. Mendelsohn
10. "Real Food for Pregnancy" by Lily Nichols
11. "Nurture" by Erica Chidi Cohen
12. "The Continuum Concept" by Jean Liedloff
13. "Simplicity Parenting" by Kim John Payne
14. "Vaccines: A Reappraisal" by Dr. Richard Moskowitz
15. "The Mama Natural Week-by-Week Guide to Pregnancy &

Childbirth" by Genevieve Howland

Websites & Blogs

1. Mama Natural – mamanatural.com
2. Wellness Mama – wellnessmama.com
3. The Holistic Mama – theholisticmama.com
4. Green Child Magazine – greenchildmagazine.com
5. Natural Baby Mama – naturalbabymama.com
6. Organic Authority – organicauthority.com
7. Earth Mama Organics – earthmamaorganics.com
8. Mothering Magazine – mothering.com
9. The Crunchy Mommy – crunchymommy.com
10. Aviva Romm, M.D. – avivaromm.com
11. The Eco-Friendly Family – eco-friendlyfamily.com
12. KellyMom – kellymom.com
13. Grist – grist.org
14. Natural Baby Care – naturalbabycare.org
15. Raising Natural Kids – raisingnaturalkids.com

Podcasts

1. The Wellness Mama Podcast
2. The Birth Hour Podcast
3. The Balanced Bites Podcast
4. The Doctor Mom Podcast
5. The Holistic Kids Show
6. The Crunchy Mom Podcast
7. Minimalist Moms Podcast
8. The Real Food RDs Podcast
9. Aviva Romm MD Podcast

10. The Healthy Moms Podcast
11. The Nourished Child Podcast
12. The Natural Birth Podcast
13. Mindful Mama Podcast
14. Unruffled Podcast
15. The Sustainable Minimalists Podcast

Documentaries

1. "The Business of Being Born"
2. "Forks Over Knives"
3. "Food, Inc."
4. "The Magic Pill"
5. "Stink!"
6. "Seed: The Untold Story"
7. "The True Cost"
8. "Vaxxed: From Cover-Up to Catastrophe"
9. "Fed Up"
10. "Inhabit: A Permaculture Perspective"
11. "That Sugar Film"
12. "What the Health"
13. "GMO OMG"
14. "Vaccines Revealed"
15. "The Milk System"

Organizations

1. La Leche League International – llli.org
2. National Vaccine Information Center – nvic.org
3. Children's Health Defense – childrenshealthdefense.org
4. Weston A. Price Foundation – westonaprice.org

5. The Holistic Moms Network – holisticmoms.org
6. EcoParents Network – ecoparents.com
7. Natural Parenting Network
8. The Environmental Working Group (EWG) – ewg.org
9. Holistic Pediatric Alliance – holisticpediatricalliance.org
10. Organic Consumers Association – organicconsumers.org
11. Generation Rescue – generationrescue.org
12. Attachment Parenting International – attachmentparenting.org
13. Natural Health Federation – thenhf.com
14. Permaculture Institute – permaculture.org
15. Herbalists Without Borders – hwbglobal.org

Natural & Eco-Friendly Products

1. Earth Mama Organics – Safe baby and mama care products.
2. Burt's Bees Baby – Organic clothing and baby care products.
3. Thrive Market – Natural and organic groceries delivered to your door.
4. Honest Company – Non-toxic baby, cleaning, and personal care products.
5. Dr. Bronner's – Organic soaps, cleaning products, and personal care items.
6. Seventh Generation – Eco-friendly cleaning and personal care products.
7. Green Toys – Safe, Eco-friendly toys made from recycled materials.
8. Ergobaby – Baby carriers that promote healthy hip development.
9. Bamboo Nature Diapers – Eco-friendly, chemical-free

diapers.

10. Grove Collaborative – Natural household and personal care products.

Educational Resources & Alternative Education

1. Wild + Free – bewildandfree.org – Resources for nature-based homeschooling and parenting.
2. Unschooling Mom2Mom – unschoolingmom2mom.com
3. Montessori for Everyone – montessoriforeveryone.com
4. Project-Based Homeschooling – projectbasedhomeschooling.com
5. Oak Meadow – oakmeadow.com – Waldorf-inspired homeschooling curriculum.
6. Khan Academy – khanacademy.org – Free online educational resources.
7. Forest Schools USA – forestschoolsusa.org – Outdoor-based education.
8. Living Montessori Now – livingmontessorinow.com
9. Simple Homeschool – simplehomeschool.net
10. Brave Writer – bravewriter.com – Creative writing for homeschoolers.
11. Growing Up Wild – growingupwild.com – Nature-based education resources.
12. Charlotte Mason Institute – charlottemasoninstitute.org
13. Waldorf Homeschoolers – waldorfhomeschoolers.com

Apps & Tools

1. Think Dirty – An app to scan products for harmful chemicals and find safer alternatives.
2. EWG's Healthy Living App – Provides ratings for food, personal care, and household products for safety and environmental impact.

Commonly Used Homeopathic Remedies and Their Uses

1. **Arnica montana** – For bruises, muscle pain, trauma, and post-surgery recovery.
2. **Aconitum napellus** – For sudden high fever, shock, or panic attacks.
3. **Belladonna** – For high fever, throbbing headaches, and ear infections.
4. **Nux vomica** – For indigestion, hangovers, irritability, and constipation.
5. **Chamomilla** – For teething pain, irritability, and colic in infants.
6. **Pulsatilla** – For colds, earaches, and mood swings (especially in children).
7. **Allium cepa** – For hay fever, runny nose, and watery eyes.
8. **Rhus toxicodendron** – For joint pain, stiffness, and rashes (like poison ivy).
9. **Bryonia** – For dry coughs, joint pain, and headaches worsened by movement.
10. **Euphrasia** – For watery eyes, hay fever, and conjunctivitis.
11. **Ignatia amara** – For grief, emotional distress, or mood

swings.

12. **Gelsemium** – For flu with fatigue, weakness, and droopy eyelids.
13. **Calcarea carbonica** – For slow development in children, teething issues, and fatigue.
14. **Hepar sulphuris** – For abscesses, infected wounds, and sensitive coughs.
15. **Apis mellifica** – For bee stings, hives, swelling, and allergic reactions.
16. **Hypericum perforatum** – For nerve pain, injuries to fingers or toes, and puncture wounds.
17. **Silicea** – For abscesses, pus-filled infections, and weak nails.
18. **Spongia tosta** – For dry, barking coughs, particularly at night.
19. **Ferrum phosphoricum** – For the early stages of colds, infections, and fevers.
20. **Natrum muriaticum** – For grief, headaches, and dry skin.
21. **Arsenicum album** – For food poisoning, diarrhea, and anxiety.
22. **Phosphorus** – For nosebleeds, respiratory infections, and bleeding issues.
23. **Causticum** – For hoarseness, loss of voice, and urinary incontinence.
24. **Mercurius solubilis** – For sore throat, swollen glands, and excessive salivation.
25. **Kali bichromicum** – For thick, sticky mucus and sinus infections.
26. **Magnesia phosphorica** – For cramping, menstrual pain, and colic.
27. **Lachesis** – For circulatory issues, left-sided complaints,

and menopausal symptoms.

28. **Sulphur** – For skin conditions like eczema, rashes, and itching.
29. **Ruta graveolens** – For sprains, tendonitis, and eye strain.
30. **Veratrum album** – For severe vomiting, diarrhea, and dehydration.

100 Herbal Remedies for Kids

1. **Chamomile** – Soothes digestive discomfort, reduces anxiety, promotes sleep.
2. **Elderberry** – Boosts immunity, especially helpful for colds and flu.
3. **Echinacea** – Strengthens the immune system to fight infections.
4. **Lavender** – Calms the mind, helps with sleep and mild skin irritations.
5. **Peppermint** – Eases digestive issues, reduces headaches, clears nasal congestion.
6. **Ginger** – Relieves nausea, aids digestion, and helps with colds.
7. **Calendula** – Heals cuts, scrapes, and skin irritations.
8. **Slippery Elm** – Soothes sore throats and aids digestion.
9. **Licorice Root** – Helps soothe coughs and sore throats.
10. **Thyme** – Fights respiratory infections and soothes coughs.
11. **Fennel** – Relieves gas and bloating, especially in babies.
12. **Lemon Balm** – Calms anxiety and promotes restful sleep.
13. **Marshmallow Root** – Soothes irritated tissues, particularly the throat and digestive tract.

14. **Rosemary** – Boosts memory and improves focus.
15. **Catnip** – Relieves colic and promotes restful sleep.
16. **Yarrow** – Reduces fever and helps with colds.
17. **Hibiscus** – Supports heart health and boosts immunity.
18. **Oregano** – Fights infections and supports respiratory health.
19. **Mullein** – Helps with respiratory issues like coughs and congestion.
20. **Stinging Nettle** – Supports overall health and reduces seasonal allergies.
21. **Red Clover** – Supports detoxification and skin health.
22. **Dandelion Root** – Supports liver function and digestion.
23. **Goldenseal** – Fights bacterial infections.
24. **Turmeric** – Anti-inflammatory, supports immune health.
25. **Raspberry Leaf** – Supports digestive health and is great for teenage girls' menstrual issues.
26. **Valerian Root** – Calms nervousness and helps with sleep.
27. **Cinnamon** – Regulates blood sugar and soothes digestive issues.
28. **Clove** – Natural pain relief for toothaches.
29. **Sage** – Soothes sore throats and digestive issues.
30. **Plantain** – Heals skin irritations and insect bites.
31. **Ginseng** – Boosts energy and strengthens the immune system.
32. **Aloe Vera** – Heals burns, cuts, and skin irritations.
33. **Comfrey** – Supports healing of broken bones and sprains.
34. **Chickweed** – Soothes skin rashes and irritations.
35. **Bilberry** – Supports eye health and improves circulation.
36. **Hawthorn** – Supports heart health and emotional balance.
37. **Holy Basil (Tulsi)** – Reduces stress and boosts immunity.
38. **Eucalyptus** – Clears nasal congestion and supports respi-

ratory health.

39. **Arnica** – Helps with bruises and muscle pain.
40. **Burdock Root** – Cleanses the blood and supports skin health.
41. **Fenugreek** – Helps with respiratory conditions and breast-feeding support.
42. **Grapefruit Seed Extract** – Fights bacterial and fungal infections.
43. **Meadowsweet** – Relieves pain and reduces fever.
44. **Licorice Root** – Soothes coughs and aids digestion.
45. **Blue Vervain** – Supports relaxation and calms anxiety.
46. **Spearmint** – Aids digestion and eases headaches.
47. **Coriander** – Supports digestion and reduces bloating.
48. **Angelica Root** – Supports respiratory health and relieves colds.
49. **Hyssop** – Clears congestion and supports lung health.
50. **Wood Betony** – Calms anxiety and improves digestion.
51. **Anise Seed** – Soothes upset stomachs and aids digestion.
52. **Sarsaparilla** – Supports skin health and detoxification.
53. **Marjoram** – Eases digestive issues and supports respiratory health.
54. **Wintergreen** – Relieves muscle aches and reduces inflammation.
55. **Red Raspberry Leaf** – Great for teenage girls' menstrual health and digestive support.
56. **Black Cohosh** – Soothes menstrual cramps and hormonal imbalances.
57. **Bayberry** – Astringent for sore throats and diarrhea.
58. **White Willow Bark** – Natural pain reliever, similar to aspirin.
59. **Cranberry** – Supports urinary tract health.

60. **Milk Thistle** – Supports liver detoxification and skin health.
61. **Astragalus** – Boosts immunity and helps fight infections.
62. **Ashwagandha** – Reduces stress and boosts overall energy.
63. **Elecampane** – Supports lung health and clears congestion.
64. **Passionflower** – Calms anxiety and promotes restful sleep.
65. **Skullcap** – Relieves nervous tension and supports emotional health.
66. **Basil** – Supports digestion and boosts immunity.
67. **Parsley** – Rich in nutrients and supports kidney health.
68. **Juniper Berries** – Supports urinary health and helps with infections.
69. **Linden Flower** – Soothes colds and fevers, promotes relaxation.
70. **Sandalwood** – Calms nerves and supports skin health.
71. **Chamomile Tea** – Calms the digestive system and helps children sleep.
72. **Rose Hips** – High in vitamin C, boosts immune health.
73. **Peppermint Tea** – Soothes digestive issues and clears congestion.
74. **Siberian Ginseng** – Boosts energy and supports immunity.
75. **Motherwort** – Calms anxiety and supports heart health.
76. **Thyme Tea** – Fights respiratory infections and soothes coughs.
77. **Cayenne Pepper** – Stimulates circulation and relieves pain.
78. **Tarragon** – Aids digestion and eases toothaches.
79. **Mugwort** – Supports digestion and calms the nervous system.
80. **Black Walnut** – Helps with parasite infections and supports digestion.
81. **Wild Yam** – Soothes cramps and supports hormonal bal-

ance.

82. **Gotu Kola** – Supports brain health and cognitive function.
83. **Birch Bark** – Reduces pain and inflammation.
84. **Barberry** – Supports liver health and digestion.
85. **Chamomile Oil** – Calms anxiety and relieves skin irritation.
86. **Dill** – Soothes digestive issues, especially in babies.
87. **Chaste Tree Berry** – Balances hormones, especially for teenage girls.
88. **Oregon Grape Root** – Supports liver function and skin health.
89. **Cornsilk** – Helps with urinary tract issues.
90. **Peppermint Oil** – Relieves headaches and eases nausea.
91. **Rosemary Oil** – Supports memory and relieves muscle pain.
92. **Feverfew** – Prevents migraines and reduces fever.
93. **St. John's Wort** – Supports mood balance and emotional health.
94. **Borage** – Supports adrenal function and reduces stress.
95. **Kava Kava** – Relieves anxiety and stress.
96. **Willow Bark** – Natural pain reliever, especially for headaches.
97. **Saffron** – Uplifts mood and improves digestion.
98. **Chrysanthemum** – Supports eye health and reduces fever.
99. **Tansy** – Helps with parasites and digestive issues.
100. **Wormwood** – Known for its anti parasitic properties.

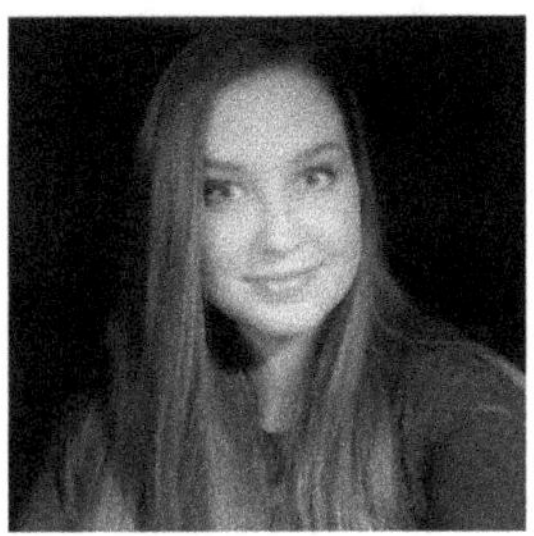

About the Author

Ashley Smith Biro is a devoted holistic health practitioner, author, and mother passionate about natural health and wellness. With years of experience in holistic practices, Ashley has dedicated her career to empowering families to make informed, balanced choices for their health. She is the founder of Fire & Ice Holistic Health and Holistic Leaders Collective,, where she provides guidance through massage therapy, holistic health consultations, and educational resources.

Drawing from her personal journey as a parent and professional experience, Ashley shares practical tips and heartfelt insights on nurturing physical, mental, and emotional well-being. Her mission is to inspire parents to foster resilience and connection in their children while building a supportive, holistic community.

Also by Ashley Smith Biro

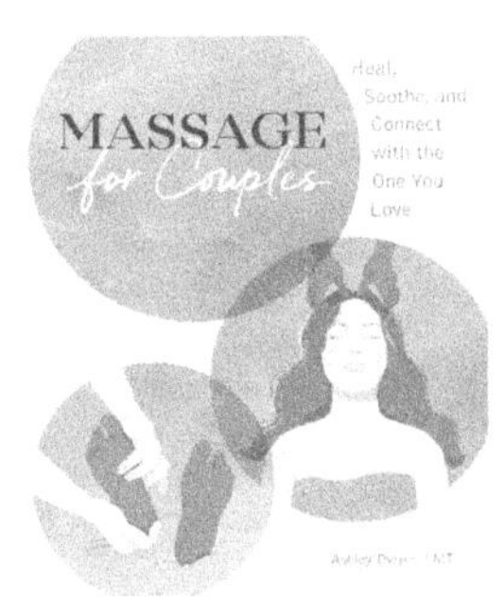

Massage for Couples

Discover a deeper connection with your partner through the healing power of massage

There's nothing like the stress-relieving, mood-lifting comfort of physical touch to bring out the best in your relationship. Whether you are helping a partner with aches and pains or looking to foster intimacy, *Massage for Couples* will teach you time-honored techniques from around the world that have made massage a staple for relaxation and relationship longevity since ancient times.

Begin by gaining confidence in using your hands to provide a healing touch. Then discover guided massage sequences to soothe, inspire, uplift, relax, or resolve a specific pain point. Support your partner's well-being and enjoy a healthy, enriching way to spend quality time together.

Inside *Massage for Couples*, you'll find:

Naturally healing together—Practice a holistic method of experiencing pleasure and providing relief from stress and fatigue.

Body wisdom—Educate yourself on some light biology and anatomy lessons that will help you refine your skills and give truly transformative, bliss-inspiring massages.

Comfort and connection—Master instructions for resolving specific aches and pains as well as tips for connecting with a partner emotionally.

Learn the healing power of touch to promote wellness and heighten intimacy with *Massage for Couples*.

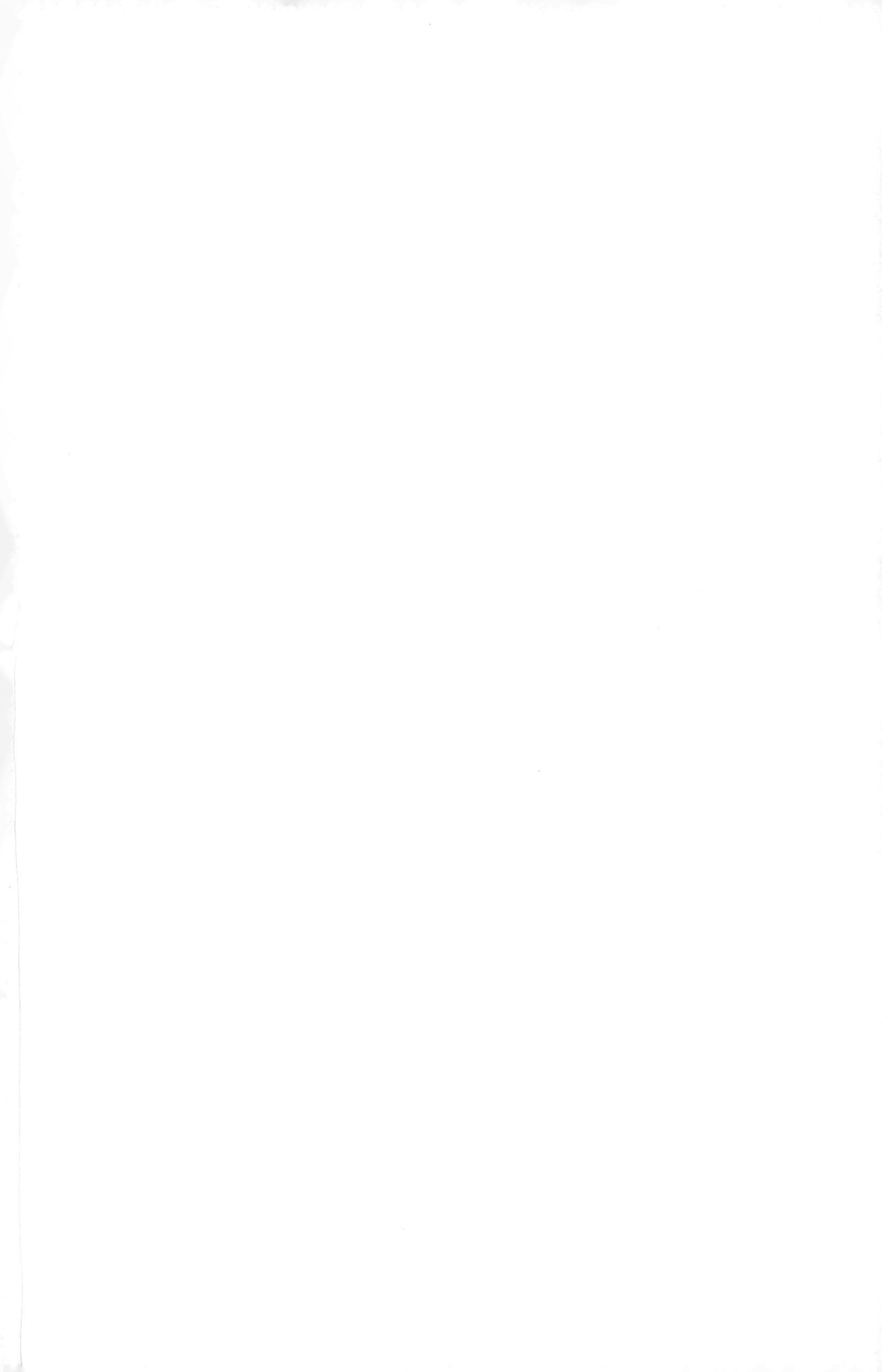

www.ingramcontent.com/pod-product-compliance
Ingram Content Group UK Ltd.
Pitfield, Milton Keynes, MK11 3LW, UK
UKHW022028190726
13853UKWH00005B/2160

9 798330 583287